HEALING
LOW BACK
PAIN

YOGA, NATUROPATHY & PHYSIOTHERAPY

ROSAMMA. T.

PREFACE

In fact the topic; "Back Pain & it's cure" is so much associated with Physical Education since the latter gives prime importance to Physical Exercises. Back pain is so common in India as well as all over the world and it's major causes are lack of proper Exercises and improper Posture. The new life style and the food habits of human beings of the present day, should be changed for getting a relief from this disease. "Yogic Practices and Naturopathic diet" have very significant role in curing even acute and chronic low back pain. The present   has focussed on the effect of "Yogic Practices, Naturopathic and Physiotherapy treatment" on low back pain patients. It has been proved that the combined treatment of Yogic Practices and Naturopathic treatment is so much beneficial for the low back pain patients. I hope that people would realize the benefit of Yoga & Naturopathy which is really cost effective in curing lower back ache in the coming days.

ROSAMMA.T

CONTENTS

LIST OF TABLES

LIST OF ILLUSTRATIONS (Photographs & Other Pictures)

LIST OF APPENDICES

Chapter i

INTRODUCTION

Chapter i

INTRODUCTION

1.1 Education, Physical Education, Health, Fitness & Physical Fitness

About Education, Rabindranath Tagore said; "The highest education is that which does not merely give us information, but makes our life in harmony with all existence".[1]

According to Bucher and Wuest,[2] Physical Education is an integral part of the total education process in a field of endeavour, which has it's aim in the development of physically, mentally, emotionally and socially fit citizens. Mathews[3] states; the primary aim of physical education is to develop a natural vitality with charactor, values and physical fitness in individuals. Lumpkin says,[4] Physical Education's objective is to develop the various organic systems of the body so as to respond in a healthful way to the increased demands placed on them.

---

[1] Dhiman.O.P., <u>Foundation of Education,</u> Atmaram and Sons, New Delhi, 1987, P.19

[2] Charles.A.Bucher, Deborach.A.Wuest, <u>Foundation of Physical Education and Sports,</u> C.V.Mosby Company, St. Louis, 1987, P.55

[3] Donald.K.Mathews; <u>Measurement of Physical Education,</u> W.B.Saunders Company, Philadelphia, 1976, P.72

[4] Angela Lumpkin; <u>Physical Education, a Contemporary Introduction,</u> C.V.Mosby Comapny, St.Louis, 1986, P.246

According to Singh, Gill and Bains, Physical Education includes all the aspects leading to all-round and total development of an individual.[5]

Planning Commission of India charter says, health is a positive state of well-being in which harmonious development of mental and physical capacities of the individual leads to enjoyment of a rich and full life.[6] According to Marley and William, health is a state of the total effective physiological and psychological functioning.[7] Steinhaus says, Health is a state of complete physical, mental and social well being and not merely the absence of diseases or infirmity".[8]

About fitness, Frost is of the view that it is a state which characterises the degree to which a person is able to function.[9] For Hezedline, Physical Fitness is the total dynamic physiological state of the individual which comprises strength, speed, endurence, flexibility and co-ordination.[10] "A healthy mind in a healthy

---

[5] Ajmer Singh, Jagtar Singh Gill, Jagdish Bains, Essentials of Physical Education, Kalyani Publishers, New Delhi, 2004, P.20

[6] Planning Commission, First Five Year Plan Charter (1950-55), Government of India, New Delhi, P.187

[7] Marley, William.P, Health and Physical Fitness, W.B.Saunders Company, New York, 1982, P.76

[8] Arthur.R.Steinhaus, Towards an understanding of Health and Physical Education, WMC Brown Company Publishers, Mississippi, 1963, P.5

[9] Reuban.B.Frost, Psychological Concepts applied to Physical Education and Coaching, Addison Wesley Publishing Company Inc, California, 1971, P.70

[10] Rex Hezedline, Fitness for Sports, The Crowood Press, Malborough, 1985, P.4

body", as Hooks [11] says. Every one has to be physically fit, if he has to discharge his duties effectively.

1.2   LOW BACK PAIN

Low Back Pain is one of the most common problems among adults, largely as a result of strained muscles or ligaments or trapped spinal nerves.[12] McRae says; Low Back Pain is one of the commonest and troublesome of compliants, it's causes are legion and an exact diagnosis is often difficult.[13] Tulder, Jellema and Poppel are of the view that Low Back Pain is the second most common pain compliant among the adult population.[14] Low Back Pain is a leading musculoskeletal compliant that contribute impairement and disability ;[15] says Cuccurullo.

---

[11] Gene Hooks, <u>Application of Weight Training to Athlets</u>, Prentice Hall INC, Englewood Cliffs, New Jersy, 1962, P.1

[12] Pilates Patricia Lamond, <u>Harmonious Body Control</u>, New Holland Publishers, London, 2002, P.11

[13] Ronald McRae, <u>Pocket Book of Orthopaedics and Fractures,</u> Churchill Livingstone, Edinburgh, 2006, P.84

[14] Van Tulder.M.W, Jellema.P., Van Poppel.M.N.M., <u>Lumbar Supports for Prevention and Treatment of low back pain,</u> (Cochrane Review), Cochrane Library Issue No.4, Oxford, 2000.

[15] Sara.J.J.Cuccurullo, <u>Physical Medicine and Rehabilitation Board Review,</u> Domos Medical Publishing, New York, 2004, P.256

White and Gorgon say "Low back pain is a common cause of disability, particularly during the productive middle years of adult life".[16] Surveys reveal that for persons younger than 45 years, mechanical Low Back Pain represents the most common cause of disability.[17]

Low Back Pain is usually caused by minor damage to the ligaments and muscles in the back.[18] It may be the result of a prolapsed or herniated disc in the spine. According to Sakamoto, Low Back Pain is one of the most prevalent complaints, the diagnosis of the mechanism or source of low back pain is therefore very challenging.[19] Low Back Pain is associated with many ergonomic stressors including lifting, carrying of heavy loads, freequent bending, and awkward postures.[20] In early disc lesions, the characteristic is aching, dependant

---

[16] Augusts .A. White, Stephan. L. Gorgon, Symposium on Diopathic Low back pain, Mosby Co, St.Louis, London, 2001, P. 82.

[17] Ronald Bodley Scott, Price's Text Book of the Practice of Medicine, The English Language Book Society and Oxford University Press, 1966, P 956.

[18] David.R.Goldmann, Complete Home Medical Guide, D.K.Publishing INC, New York, 1999, PP.383-384

[19] Sakamoto.A., Low Back Pain and it's Remedies, Journal of Nippon Medical School, Tokyo,2002,Dec;69(6):588-92.

[20] The World Health Report 2002, World Health Organization (Reducing Risks, Promoting Healthy Life), Genewa, Switzerland, 2002, P.76

on how much the patient exerts his back, which is the cause of ordinary Low Back Pain.[21]

Low back Pain and Posture

Cyriax says, originally the Lumbar spine needed to be strong in resisting strains; now it must resist repeated flexions. Now man can stand upright, unwanted compression aggravates the stress.[22] Poor posture is, when it is inefficient, that is when it fails to serve the purpose for which it was designed or if an unnecessary amount of muscular effort is used to maintain it.[23] Tall slim people with willowy backs are said to be especially prone to acute low back strains, as are those in sedentary occupations.[24] 80 - 90% of the people who suffer from Low Back Pain in do so, because of the improper care of their back due to bad habits of posture.[25]

---

[21] Weinstein.S.L., Buck Walter.J.A. (ed), <u>Tureck's Orthopaedics-Principles and their applications</u> (5th edn), J.B.Lippincott Company, Philadelphia, 1994, P.126

[22] James Cyriax; <u>Text book of Orthopaedic Medicine (Diagnosis of soft tissue lesions)</u>, BAILLIERE TINDALL, London, 1981, P. 222.

[23] Dena Gardiner.M., <u>The Principles of Exercise Therapy</u>, C.B.S.Publishers and Distributors, New Delhi, 1990, P.248

[24] Khosla.S.N., <u>Every Man's guide to perfect health</u>, PEACOCK BOOKS, New Delhi, 2006, P.420

[25] Porter Richard.W., <u>Management of Back Pain</u> (2nd edn), Churchill Livingstone, Edinburgh, 1993, P.234

Acute and Chronic Low Back Pain

If the pain lasts for less than three months, it is called acute back pain, If the problem goes on for longer, then it is is known as chronic back pain.[26] In chronic cases there is often a long history of intermittent low back pain over a number of years.[27] A practical approach to the management of Low Back Pain is to consider acute and chronic presentations separately.[28] Risk factors include; overweight, restricted spinal mobility, poor self rated health, minimal physical activity etc.

Back pain is of two types; an acute some times severe pain, well localized to the midline over a restricted region of the spine, which disappears over a period of weeks and a much more chronic, diffusing, aching pain.[29]

---

[26] Ellis.R.M, Back Pain, <u>British Medical Journal</u>, 310 (6989), 1220, 1995.

[27] Kirkaldy-Willis.WH, Burton.CV (eds), <u>Managing Low Back Pain,</u> (3rd ed), Churchill Livingstone, New York, 1992, P.348

[28] Dennis.L.Kasper, Anthoni.S.Fouci, Dan.L.Longo, <u>Harrisons's Principles of Internal Medicine,</u> 16th edn, Mcgraw-Hill Medical publishing Division, New York, 2005, PP.100-101

[29] Pope.M.H., Frymoer.J.W., Anderson.G.,(eds) <u>Occupational Low back pain</u>, Praeger Press, New York, 1984, P.437

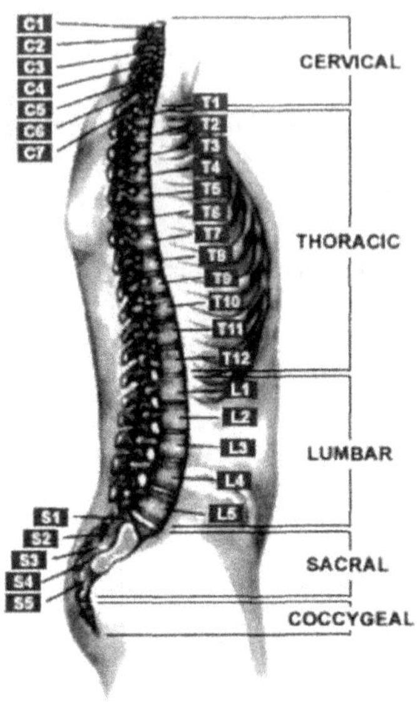

The Spine (lateral view)

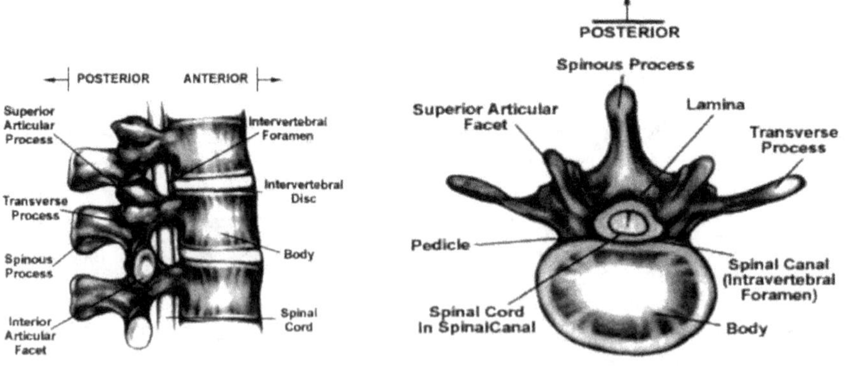

Lumbar Vertebrae (lateral view)   **Lumbar Vertebra** (top view)

How the Back Works

The spine is made up of many small bones called vertebrae. These are separated by discs, which allow the spine to bend. This structure of vertebrae and discs is and discs is supported along its length by muscles and ligaments. The spinal cord threads through the centre of each vertebra, carrying nerves from the brain to the rest of the body.[30] A healthy Spine in standing position is S shaped with an inward curve at the lower end; lordosis. Bad posture when sitting and squatting exxagerates this curve leading to a proplapsed disc or osteoarthritis of the spine.[31]

1.2.1 Classification of Low Back Pain

Back specialists understand low back problems by dividing the same in to different categories; mechanical low back pain and compressive low back pain.[32]

Mechanical Back Pain

Mechanical pain often called back strain because it is linked with the "the mechanics" of the spine which occurs when injury to the spine's discs, facet

---

[30] John Tanner, <u>Your Guide to Back Pain,</u> Hodder Arnold Publishers, London, 2005, P.37

[31] Susan Clark,<u>What really works in Natural Health.</u>, Bentham Press, London, 2004, P.193

[32] David.J.Dandy, Dennis.J.Edwards, <u>Essentials of Orthopaedics and Trauma,</u> Churchill Living stone, Edinburgh,1998, P 425

joints, ligaments, or muscles results in inflammation.[33] Causes of mechanical Low Back Pain generally are attributed to an acute traumatic event but also may include cumulative trauma.[34] Low Back Pain at night unrelieved by rest, suggests the posibility of malignancy; either vertebral body metastasis or a quada equina.[35]

Most common causes of Low Back Pain are injuries, stress resulting in musculoskeletal disorders, infections, Osteoarthritis, rheumatoid arthritis, spinal stenosis, tumours and congenital disorders. Low Back Pain is commoner in women who have had several pregnancies.[36] Abnormalities of a facet joint and disc prolapse can both cause sciatica, resulting from pressure on a sciatic nerve root as it leaves the spinal cord. [37] In Lumbago type low back pain, the patient is suddenly seized with agonizing, in the lumbar region of the spine while stooping, lifting or turning.[38] In Scoliosis type mechanical low back pain the

---

[33] Lawrence.M.Tierney, Steephen.J.Mcphee, Maxine.A.Papadakis, Current Medical Diagnosis & Treatment, Lange Medical Books/ McGraw Hill, New York, 2004, P.788

[34] Brinker.MR, Miller.M., Fundamentals of Orthopaedics, W.B.Saunders, Philadelphia, 1999, P.196

[35] Rowlingson.J.C, Keifer.R.B, Low Back Pain, in Ashburn.M.A, Rice.L.J.,(editors),The Management of Pain, Churchill Living Stone, New York, 1998, P.249

[36] Cole.A.J, Herring .S.A, The Low back Pain; A practical guide for Primary care Clinician, Hanley and Belfus, Philadelphia, 1997, P.38

[37] Louise.L.Hay, Heal Your Body, Hay House (U.K.) Ltd, London, 1982, P.75

[38] John CrawFord Adams, David.L.Hamblen, Out line of Orthopaedics, Churchill Livingstone, London, 2001, P.205

deformity is characterized by lateral curvature and vertebral rotation.[39] The Spina bifida type mechanical low back pain is associated with mal-development of the spinal cord and the membranes.[40]

Compressive Back Pain

Compressive pain is the result of pressure on the spinal cord, or nerves that leave the spine.[41] If an intervertebral disc herniates and pushes in to the spinal canal, it can cause pain. Sciatica which is a type of compressive pain radiates down the back of the thigh and calf. Degenerative arthritis and Disc prolapse are the causes.[42]

Arthritis Pain

Arthritis of the spine usually refers to a condition where there is inflammation of the facet joints between the vertebrae.[43] Ageing changes in the structures of the spine can also cause Low back pain.[44] Lumbar Spondylosis or

---

[39] Hugo Keim, Robert Hensinger, Spinal Deformities, Scoliosis and Khyphosis, Clinical Symposia, Vol.41, No.4, CIBA-GEIGY Corp.1989, PP.23-24

[40] Maheswari.J, Essential Orthopaedics, Mehtha Publishers, New Delhi, 1993, P.210.

[41] Russel.R.C.G., Norman.S.Williams, Christopher.J.K.Bulstrode, Baily & Love's Short Practice of Surgery, Arnold Publishers, London, 2004, P.564.

[42] Herrlngs.3, Weinstein.3., Assessment and Neurological Management of Athletic low back injury, in Nocholas.J., Herschman.F., The Lower extremity and Spine in Sports Medicine, Mosby Co, St.Louis, 1995, P.153

[43] The British Medical Association, Complete Family Health Encyclopaedia, Dorling Kindersley Ltd, London, 1993, P.136

[44] The Readers Digest Association Limited, Family Guide to Alternative Medicine, London, 1991, P.58

11

"wear and tear of the spine" is another reason for low back pain.[45] Ankylosing spondylitis begins as vague low back pain after periods of inactivity such as overnight sleep and later on develops to severe pain. [46] Loss of muscle strength is a feature of Ankylosing Spondylitis.[47] Muscles weaken owing to postural deformity and inactivity and this causes pain. Osteoarthritis can come from a single injury that damages the joint or from a lifetime of overuse of different joints that damage the joint a little bit.[48] Facet joint syndrome which is one of the reason for low back pain is caused by a combination of aging, pressure overload of the facet joints and injury.[49] Spines that show indications of spondylosis, also often show osteoarthritic changes in the corresponding facet joints and thus results in low back pain.[50] Radiculopathy is a "pinched nerve" in the spine which also can causes low back pain.[51]

---

[45] Guiot.B.H., Fessler.R.G., Molecular Biology of Degenerative Disc Diseases, Neuorosurgery, 2000, 47 (5): 1034

[46] Paul Anand, Mehta.A.B, Siddharth.N.Shah, Sainani.G.S, Viswanathan.M, A.P.I.Text Book of Medicine, Association of Physicians of India, Bombay, 1988, P.1055

[47] Cooper.R., Freemont.A., Fitzmaurice.R., Paraspinal Muscle Fibrosis, a specific pathological component in Ankylosing Spondylitis, Annals of Rheumatic Diseases., 1991, 50 (11): 755-759

[48] Rowlingson.J.C, Keifer.R.B, Low Back Pain, In Ashburn.M.A, Rice.L.J.,(editors), The Management of Pain, Churchill Living Stone, New York, 1998, P.187

[49] Adams.M.A., Hutton.W.C., The Mechanical Function of the Lumbar Apophyseal joints, Spine, 2002 8 (3): 327 – 30

[50] Dolan.P., Adams.M.A., Recent Advances in Lumbar Spinal mechanics and their significance in Modelling, Clinical Biomechanics, 2001, 16 Suppl. 1: s8 – s16

[51] Brown.DE, Neumann.RD, Orthopaedic Secrets, 2nd ed., Hanley & Belfus, Philadelphia, 1999, P.319

Spinal stenosis which is the narrowing of a portion of the spinal canal also results in low back pain.[52] Spinal stenosis usually occurs in older people after years of wear and tear of the spine. Injuries, infections, or tumours are also the causes. [53] Segmental Stenosis; the narrowing of the spinal canal in a segmented area also results in low back pain.[54] Discogenic pain caused by a damaged intervertebral disc usually causes pain felt in the lower back.[55] Some intervertebral discs begin to bulge as a part of the ageing process, and this ultimately results in low back pain.[56]

The repeated daily stresses and minor injuries can add up and begin to affect the discs in the spine and causes degeneration which also causes low back pain.[57] When there is too much movement between two vertebrae, the excess movement of vertebrae causes irritation of nerve roots and thus causes low back pain.[58] Sprain, Strain, Vertebral fractures and Disc protrusion are examples of

---

[52] Jamie.A.Alvarez, Spinal Stenosis and Low back pain, American Family Physician, April 15, 1998, P.28

[53] Geetha Sunder, A to Z of BONE, MUSCLE & JOINT Diseases, Macmillen India Ltd, 2005, P.53

[54] Paul.N.Beeson, Walsh Mc Dermott, Cecil-Loeb Text Book of Medicine, W.B.Saunders Company, Philadelphia, 1971, P.1862.

[55] Stuart Porter, Tidy's Physiotherapy, Butter worth-Heinemann Publishers, Oxford, 2003, P.116

[56] Parveen Kumar, Michael Clark, Kumar & Clark Clinical Medicinem, W.B.Saunders, Edinburgh, 2002, P.523

[57] Waddell.G., A New Clinical Model for the Treatment of Low Back Pain, Spine 12:632, 1987.

traumatic causes which results in low back pain.[59] Vertebral fractures which occur either by direct violence or indirectly leads to low back pain.[60] Disc protrusion, later leads to it's prolapse also causes low back pain. [61] Prolapse of the nucleus through the capsule-prolapsed intervertebral disc, may cause pressure on adjacent nerve roots, leading to low back pain.[62] Spinal tuberculosis is a common cause of persistant low back pain.[63]

Osteoporotic bones are brittle and therefore fracture easily. Each fracture leads to sudden onset of low back pain which is severe. [64] Osteoporosis, an age related reduction in bone mass and density which ultimately increases the person's susceptibility to fractures results in low back pain.[65] Osteoporosis is likely to develop in individuals with spinal cord injuries.[66] Calcium deficiency

---

[58] Paulson.S.(editor), <u>Santa Clara Valley Medical Center Spinal cord injury Home Manual,</u> edn.3., Santa Clara valley Medical Center, 1994, P.39

[59] Moore.J.et al, <u>The Back Pain Help Book</u>, Perseus Books Group, Cambridge, 1999, P.41

[60] Rockwood.C.A., Green.D.P. (eds), <u>Fractures in Adults</u>, Vol.1&2 (2nd edn), J.B.Lippincett, Philadelphia, 1984, P.217

[61] Bailey and Love, <u>A short Practice of Surgery</u>, Lewis Publishers, London, 1960, P. 406.

[62] Evelyn.C.Pearce, <u>Anatomy and Physiology for Nurses</u>, Oxford University Press, Culcutta, 1978, P.87

[63] Robert.L.Bratton, <u>American Family Physicians</u>, Vol.60: No.8, Nov.15, 1999, P.37

[64] Sharon Walker, <u>Essential Health for Women</u>, Parragon Publishing, Bristol, 1997, P.22

[65] Manu.V.Chakravarthy, Frank.W.Booth, <u>Exercise,</u> Hanley & Belfus Publishers, Philadelphia, 2003, P.272

[66] Mennel.J.M., <u>Back Pain</u>, Little Brown & Co, Boston, 1960, P.49

may lead to Osteoporosis or Bone shrinking and weakening in elderly women.[67] Osteoporosis is more common in women than men.[68] Osteoporosis occurs when resorption exceeds bone formation.[69] Immobilized patients can lose up to 40% of their original bone mineral density in one year.[70] People who are overweight greatly increase their risk of suffering low back pain and sciatica.[71] Overweight not only imposes an additional strain on the lower back, it may cause the individual to adopt a poor posture.[72] Under Exercise is an important factor in causing low back pain, because weakened muscles could not tolerate sudden strain at the back.[73]

Other Causes of Low back pain

Smoking has been shown to result in the necrosis of the nucleus pulposes as well as hypertrophy, which ultimately leads to low back pain.[74] "Trigger

---

[67] Charles.L.MEF JR. (edited by), Fitness, Health & Nutrition, Life Time Books, Amsterdam, 1987, P.127

[68] O'Neill.T.W.,Varlow.J., Cooper.C., Differences in vertebral deformity indices between three European populations, Journal of Bone Mineral Research, 1993, 8 (suppl .1): S149

[69] Chow.J.W, , Exercise and Sports Science Review, 28: 185, 2000.

[70] Leblance.A.D, Schneider.V.S, Evan.H.J., Bone Mineral loss and Recovery after 17 weeks of Bed Rest, Journal of Bone and Mineral Research, 5:843 – 850, 1990.

[71] Donald Norfolk, Conquering Back Pain, Blandford Press, London, 1997, PP.19-20.

[72] Jayson.M.V.I., Looking after Your Back, Jaico Publishing House, Bombay,1990, P.30

[73] Harrison.H.Clark, David.H.Clark, Developmental and Adapted Physical Education, Prentice Hall, Englewood Cliffs, New Jersy, 1978, P.261

[74] Uematsu.Y., Matuzaki.H., Effects of Nicotine on the Intervetebral Disc, an experimental study, Journal of Orthopaedic Science, 2001, 6 (2): 177 -178

points" which are nodules of degenerated muscle tissue that can literally trigger pain and spasm are found in the lower back muscles.[75] Neural tension which may be caused by lateral disc herniation, nerve root adhesions or vertebral infringement, also results in causes low back pain.[76] The multiple structures and elements of the lumber spine (L4-L5 and L5-S1) are suspected to have a role in producing mechanical Low Back Pain.[77]

Chemical causes play a role in the production of mechanical Low Back Pain.[78] The enzyme; phospholipase A2 (PLA2), may act directly on neural tissue, or it may be the orchestrator of a complex inflammatory response that manifests as Low Back Pain.

Low back strain in sports activities happens from a sudden extension contraction on an overloaded and under-developed spine, which results in low back pain.[79] Waddell asserts and says that, "social class" is probably the strongest personal predictor of incurring low back trouble.[80] Coste.J., et al have

---

[75] Alexander Melleby, <u>Six Weeks to a Healthy Back</u>, Sheldon Press, London, 1990, P.98.

[76] Cailliet.R., <u>Low Back Pain</u>, edn.3, F.A.Davis Publishers, Philadelphia, 1995, P.23

[77] Hardy.R.W., (ed), <u>Lumbar Disc Disease</u> (2nd edn.), Raven Press, New York, 1993, P.59

[78] Melnik.M.S., Saunders.R., Saunders.H.D., <u>Self Help Manual for Managing Back Pain</u>, Bloomington.M.N, 1989

[79] William.E.Prentice, <u>Arnheim's Principles of Athletic Training</u>, McGraw Hill International Edition, New York, 2006, PP.849-850

[80] Waddell.G., <u>The Back Pain Revolution</u>, Churchill Livingstone, New York, 1998, P.37

studied the Psychological involvement in low back pain.[81] A psychiatric disorder, according to the DSM-III criteria (axis I) was found in 41% of the subjects under study. Strengthening of the Immune System is very much effective in preventing low back pain which is caused due to diseases like Tuberculosis, as Candace Pert said.[82]

Aggarwal [83] says; sitting using the errect chair, standing with the individual's back flat, using proper foot wear, regular exercises, correcting body posture while driving the car or operating the computer, lifting heavy objects in the proper way and using good mattress arc some of the common measures by which low back pain could be prevented.

1.3 YOGA

The word Yoga derives from the root *"Yuj"* which means 'to yoke', 'to master', 'to control'.Yoga is the fact of yoking; of placing under the yoke, of mastering. For this reason, the following 'Sutra';***"YOGAS CITTAVRTTI NIRODHAH"***, defines yoga as the restraint of the mental processes.[84] The way

---

[81] Coste.J., Paolaggi.J.B., Spira.A ., Psychological Involvement in Low Back Pain, Spine, 1992 Sept.17 (9) 1028-37

[82] Candace Pert, Molecules of Emotion, Why You Feel the Way You Feel, Scribner Publishers, New York, 1997, P.181

[83] Aggarwal.B.S., Bed Room Exercises for Busy People, Rupa & Co, New Delhi, 2006, P.24

[84] Fernando Tola, Carmen Dragonetti, The Yoga Sutras of Pathanjali, Motilal Banarsidass Publishers, New Delhi, 1991, P.1.

to realize and experience it (the union of Atman and the self-hood), is to make the mind absolutely pure.[85] Yoga has also been described as wisdom in work or skillful living amongst activities, harmony and moderation.[86] Out of that yoga practice that the perfection in knowledge-of-the diffussion comes about. And so it is said by the teacher(s); *"Yogas tattva-jnane-rtha"* means, 'Yoga is for the purpose of knowledge of truth'.[87] The goal of yogic life is truely infinite with vistas of achievement which are so vast that we can't even comprehend them.[88]

Kaur says, Yoga bind together all the various parts of ourselves, often thought of as body, mind and spirit.[89] Cameron says; Yoga creates path ways in individual's consciousness through which creative and healing forces can operate.[90] When freed from obscurations by impurity, the sattva of the thinking substance, the essence of which is light, has a pellucid steady flow and this is the clearness of mind and then the yogin gains the internal undisturbed calm.[91]

---

[85] Atmananda Swamy, The Four Yogas, Bharatiya Vidhyabhavan, Bombay, 1966, P.205

[86] Iyenkar.B.K.S., Light on Yoga, Harper Collins Publishers (India), New Delhi, 2006, P.20.

[87] Trevor Leggett, On the Yoga Sutras, Motilal Banasidass Publishers, *New* Delhi, 1992, P.257.

[88] Thaimni.I.K, Glimpses in to the Psychology of Yoga, The Theosophical Publishing House, Adayar, Madras, 1973, P.11

[89] Shakta Kaur Khalsa, Yoga for Women, Dorling Kindersley Ltd, London, 2002, P.13
[90] Julie Cameron, The Artist's Way, J.P.Tarcher/ Putnam Publishers, New York, 1992, P.xiii

[91] James Haughton Woods, The Yoga-System of Patanjali, (Harward Oriental Series), Banarsidass Publishers, New Delhi, 1966, P.93

Vedanta Swami [92] says; that if one wants to engage in yoga, he should gratify the senses moderately and keep his life as free from anxiety. According to Santhi Dharmanantha;[93] Yoga provides perfection, peace and mental pleasure. A powerful antidote to the stresses of the modern life, Yoga aims at uniting the body, mind and spirit for health and fulfillment.[94]

According to Bhagavat Gita,[95] the practice of Yoga fixes the mind on God, thereby giving complete peace to the soul. Frawley [96] says, Yoga represents the higher spiritual heritage that we all hold deep within our hearts. It's methods and ideas are relevent to every one. According to Thorpe [97] yoga is as profound a science as exist, for integrating the mind, body and spirit in to a harmonious whole. Aurobindo [98] says; the true objective of Yoga can be accomplished when the conscious Yoga in man becomes, like the sub conscious Yoga in nature.

---

[92] Bhakthi Vedanta Swami Prabhupade, <u>The Perfection of Yoga,</u> The Bhakthi Vedanta Book Trust, Bombay, 1972, P.22

[93] Santhi Dharmanantha Saraswathi Swamy, <u>The Holistic Yoga,</u> Sree Kunj Sathbhavan Munch, New Delhi, 2006, P.12.

[94] Mira Mehtha, <u>How to use Yoga,</u> Annes Publishing Ltd, Bombay, 1994, P.7

[95] Satya Pal, <u>Yogasanas and Sadhana,</u> Family Books Pvt.Ltd, New Delhi, 1998, P.2

[96] David Frawley, Sandra Summerfield Kozak, <u>Yoga for Your Type,</u> Lotus Press, New York, 2001, P. 4

[97] Kumar Anish, <u>Gopi Formula (The art of Creating Health & Fitness),</u> Sahyog Ventures Pvt. Ltd, Bangalore, 2005, P.83

[98] Sri Aurobindo, <u>The Synthesis of Yoga,</u> Sri Aurobindo Ashram, Pondicherry,1984, P.4

Jung[99] is of the view that there is reason for yoga to have many adherents. It offers not only the much-sought way, but also a philosophy of unrivalled profundity. Githananda [100] says ,Yoga is a positive way of maintaining physical up keep, mental alertness and spiritual attainment.

Ashtanga Yoga, Classical Yoga and Integral Yoga

The eight fold system of Yoga (Ashtanga Yoga) includes Yama, Niyama, Asana, Pranayama, Pratyahara, Dharana, Dhyana and Samadhi. He who practice Ashtanga Yoga with patience, attains physical health and **mental peace.**[101] Classical Yoga which is presented in the context of Patanjali's "Yoga Sutras" incorporates the study of the text, the source of the teachings, and adapts to the individual with many varieties of practices beyond asanas. [102] Integral Yoga, which is a spiritual based yoga that clearly leads to meditation practice through poses taken to the extremes of flexibility.[103] There are many benefits to Yoga.

---

[99] Jung.C.G., "Yoga and the West"- in Psychology and the East, R.F.C.Hulltrans, Princeton.N.J, Princeton University Press,1978, P.81.

[100] Geethananda Swami, Meenakshi Bhavani, Yoga is a call to life- No away from life, Yoga Life :20 (Dec.1989), P.6

[101] Sudharsan Kumar Biala, Yoga for Better living and Self Realization, Kalyani Publishers, New Delhi 1999, P.36.

[102] Sree Baba Haridas, Ashtanga Yoga Primer, Sree Rama publishing, Santa Cruz, Bombay, 1981, P.41

[103] Satchitanada Swamy, Integral Yoga-Hatha, Henry Holt and Co, New York, 1970, P.17

Yoga exercises, that maintain the suppleness, which might be a factor in extending the life-span.[104]

1.3.1 Hatha Yoga

Hatha Yoga [105] represents asanas and pranayama, steps three and four of Patanjali's eight limbs. Hatha yoga seeks to balance the body with the mind. Hatha yoga[106] by it's numerous asanas, cures the body of that restlessness, a sign of it's inability to contain without working them off in action. The process of Hatha yoga is first a system of postures, which sets the body in a position in which it can stay undisturbed far as long as one wants.[107] Hatha Yoga limbers the joints and improves blood circulation through exercises, develops muscular tone through asanas and breathing exercises.[108] *"Yoga Sutra" states the process of asana and pranayama and the experiences that will arise, when it is practiced in the systematic approach.*[109] According to Kuvalayananda and Digambarji, those who are purified by pranayama, reach the supreme goal.[110]

---

[104] Paramahansa Yoganada, <u>Autobiography of a Yogi</u>, Self Realization Fellowship, Los Angeles, 1998, P.13

[105] Mukthibodhananda Swamy, <u>Hatha Yoga Pradipika,</u> Bihar school of Yoga, Munger, 1985, Chap.1

[106] Saraswathy Mukthibodhananda Swamy, <u>Hatha Yoga,</u> Bihar School of Yoga, Munger, Bihar, 1977, P.29.

[107] Pandit.M.P., <u>The Yoga of Knowledge (Based on Sri Aurobindo's Synthesis of Yoga)</u>, New Age Books, New Delhi, 2002, P.261

[108] Joan Harrington, <u>Physiological and Psychological Effects of Hatha Yoga</u>, A review of Literature, Research Bullettin, Himalayan Institute, Honesdale, 1983, PP.38-39

1.3.2 ASANA

"Asanathah Sukham hride nimajjathi" means, one who is established in a comfortable posture while concentrating on the inner self, becomes immersed in the Heart's ocean of Bliss.[111] Patanjali Maharshi defines asana as "Sthira sukhamasan",[112] means any steady comfortable posture is asana. The aim of yogasanas is mainly to regulate the proper activities of all the internal organs and glands to affect the nevous system.[113] Yogasanas aid the performance of the individual in relieving from tension, strengthen and tone the muscles, flexible and elastic.[114] Yogasana is a scientific process which gives sufficient exercise to the internal organs of the body, by which an individual can maintain good health.[115] Asanas are designed to conserve the energies and transform them to subtle form of vital and mental energies and aiding in calming down the mind.

---

[109] Mukunda Stiles, <u>Structural Yoga Therapy,</u> GoodWill Publishing House, New Delhi, 2002, P.13

[110] Kuvalayananda Swamy, Digambarji Swamy, Kokaje.P.R.G, <u>Vasishta Samhita,</u> Kaivalyadhama publishers, Lonovala, 1969, chapt.iii, sutras; 20-21.

[111] Jaideva Singh, <u>Siva Sutras; The Yoga of Supreme Identity,</u> Motilal Banarsidas Publishers, New Delhi, 1979, P.163.

[112] Sivananda Saraswathi Swami, <u>Practice of Yoga</u> (First vol.), Himalayan Yoga series, as quoted by Vinayakom.P.K., in ' <u>My magazine of India</u>', Madras, 1936, P.90

[113] Indira Devi, <u>YOGA, The Technique of Health and Happiness,</u> Jaico Publishing House, Bombay, 1970, P.20.

[114] Bugene.S.Rowles, <u>Yoga for Beauty and Health,</u> Parker Publishing Company, New York, 1967, P.19

[115] Ajmer Singh, Jagdish Bains, Jagtar Singh Gill, <u>Essentials of Physical Education,</u> Kalyani Publishers, New Delhi, 2003, P.523

[116] In Yoga, by way of asana, the individual can plug into the healing energy that is naturally available within the individual.[117] By performing asanas, the sadhaka first gains complete equillibrium of the body, mind and spirit.[118]Asanas are not movements but postures to be developed and held; most are relaxing rather than demanding effort; refreshing rather than fatiguing.[119] Asana is used to cannote different postures, which mostly involve bending and stretching of the trunk of the body and serve to keep it supple.[120]

The asanas are beneficial in overcoming certain defects in the physical body. The idea of different asanas is to gain control over the body.[121] It is true that many asanas resemble certain postures, but both are not the same.[122] In asanas attempts are made at oneness and togetherness. Most of the practices like asanas and pranayama are of a purely physical nature and when divorced from the higher and essential teaching of yoga, reduce their system to a science of

---

[116] YOGA; Asanas, Pranayama, Mudras and Kriyas, Vivekananda Kendra Publications, Madras, 1977, P.2

[117] Emma Mitchell, Boost Your Body's Energy, Duncan Baird Publishers, London, 1998, P.19

[118] Narendra.H.R., Yoga – It's Basis and Applications, Sree Vivekandanda Yoga Prakashan, Bangalore, 2000, P.39

[119] James Hevltt, The Complete Yoga Book, Rider & Company, London, 1985, P.20

[120] Earnest Wood, YOGA, Penguin Books, Middlesex, U.K., 1959, P.106

[121] Abhedhanda Swami, Yoga Psychology, Ramakrishna Vedanta Mutt, Calcutta, 1967, P.24

[122] Gore.M.M., Anatomy and Physiology of Yoga Practices, Kanchan Prakashan, Lonovala, 1988, PP. 61-62.

physical culture.[123] Yogasanas bring about equal distribution of the "prana" (vital force) throughout the body in the desired proportion for the normal state.[124] Many are the benefits of asanas. It depends, on the degree of perfection achieved and on the areas of the 'body' which are being stimulated.[125] Asanas are said to remove diseases and facilitates concentration.[126] In asanas, nerve centers are activized which control the irregularities in the body.

Yogasanas activate the endocrine glands which secrete enzymes and hormones which are essential for the proper functioning of the body and rejuvenate the entire systems of the human body.[127] Similar to Yoga tradition, in western terms, there are physical, physiological, intellectual, emotional and spiritual dimentions to human life. Yoga literally has tools to work on all of these levels.[128] In Yogic practices, there is static contraction, in which the muscles are under a stretch or tension without causing repeated movements. Yoga involves exercises of skeletal and deep seated smooth muscles of the

---

[123] Thaimni.I.K., The Science of Yoga, The Theosophical Publishing House, Adayar, Madras, 1974, P.111

[124] Chidhananda Swamy, The Philosophy, Psychology and Practice of Yoga, The Divine Life Society, Tehri, Uttar Pradesh, 1991, P.106

[125] Pranavananda Yogi, PURE YOGA, Motilal Banarsidass Publishers, New Delhi, 1992, P.60

[126] Srinivasa Iyenkar, The Hathayoga Pradeepika of Svatmarama, The Adayar Library and Research Center, Madras, 1933, P.11

[127] Govindhan Nair (Yogacharya), Yoga Vidhya, D.C.Books, Kottayam, Kerala, 1982, P.34

[128] Vishnu Devanada Swamy, Complete Illustrated Book of Yoga, Three Rivers Press, New York, 1988, P.18

body.[129] Yoga brings balanced utilization of time, mental faculties and object of sense organs.[130]

1.3.3 Pranayama

Yogic breathing is 'pranayama'. Pranayama consists of various ways of inhaling, exhaling and retention of prana; the vital life force.[131] In inhalation, oxygen enters the body and triggers off the transformation of nutrients in to fuel. In exhalation carbon dioxide is eliminated from the body. Presence of oxygen purifies the blood streams and helps invigorate each cell.[132] The aim of asana is to release mental tensions by dealing with them on the physical level, acting somato-physically through the body to mind.[133] According to Patanjali's Yoga Sutra, asanas are regarded as an aid to breath control.[134] Yogic practices have been found to contribute flexibility, according to Gharote. [135]

---

[129] Joshi.K.S., <u>Yoga in Daily Life</u>, Hind Pocket Books (P) Ltd, New Delhi, 1998, P.54

[130] Sharma.R.K., Bhagvan Dash.V., <u>Agnivesh's Charaka Samhita,"Quest for Logevity"</u>, Chow Khamba Sanskrit series office, Varanasi, 1976, PP.39-40

[131] Sreekumar.J.P., <u>Simple Yoga</u>, Yoga Brotherhood, Madras, 1960. P.33

[132] Kuvalayananda Swamy, <u>Pranayama</u>, The S.K.Y.Foundation, Philadelphia, 1978, P.113.

[133] Satyananda Saraswathy Swami, <u>Asana, Pranayama, Mudra, Bandhan</u>, Bihar School of Yoga, Munger, Bihar, 1999, P.37

[134] Surendranath DasGupta, <u>Yoga as Philosophy and Religion,</u> Motilal Banarsidass Publishers, New Delhi, 1973, P.136

[135] Gharote.M.L.,Yoga Therapy – It's scope and limitations, <u>Journal of Research and Education in Indian Medicine</u>, 1982, 1.2.P 37

Stretching in Yoga allows muscles to relax and receive increasesd blood flow and oxygen. When injury or imbalanced physical activity hinders a joint's mobility,. other joints make postural compensations.[136] In asanas the body gets flexibility and energy. The life-force flows more freely throughout the body, increasing the sense of vitality.[137] The skeletal structure is grounded and brought in to a better alignment, the nervous system perceives this stability and allows the muscles to release unnecessary tension. According to "Pathanjali" an asana is that body posture which confirms to steadiness, but at the same time, pleasant and comfortable.[138] Yogasanas help to change our attitude towards "stress". It brings oxygen and energy to cells, cleans the body by eliminating waste products and toxins.[139]

1.3.4 Therapeutic Effects of Yoga

Yogasanas are biophysio-psychological poses through which we build up many "Dams" in side our body. Blood and energy are brought to these "Dams" which then open very gradually, allowing the organs to absorb fresh healing blood and energy. When a part of the body is affected by disease, it loses it's

---

[136] Jean Couch, In defence of Stretching, <u>Yoga Journal</u>, July/Aug.1983, PP.11-12

[137] NOA BELLING, <u>Yoga: A Union of Mind and Body</u>, New Holland Publishers, London, 2002, P.17

[138] Datey.K.K., Gharote.M.L., Soli Parri; <u>Yoga and Your Heart</u>, Jaico Publishing House, Bombay, 1983, P.94

[139] Andreran Lysebath; <u>Yoga self taught</u>, Tarang Paper Back, New Delhi,1987, P.17

sensitivity. During the practice of therapeutic asanas, energy from these "Dams" flows to the affected area, allowing the healing process to begin.[140] Yogasanas are effective in throwing out the body waste and in activating the endocrine glands, on the proper functioning of which depends human health.[141] Friedeberger says,[142] Yogasanas work systematically on the muscles and joints to develop not just suppleness, but also strength, stamina,and resistance. Yoga exercises the skeletal as well as the deep seated smooth muscles of the body.[143] Yoga practices are curative measure against many ailments. Ancient Yogis formulated a therapy of yoga, to enable the system of the body to function as effectively as posible, both preventing and curing diseases.[144] Yogic perspective is to consider all pain as having it's source in a lack of understanding of ourselves. When changes to the body occurs, the body reacts in different ways. Here constant and regular Yoga practice can make difference.[145] According to Yoga any kind of mental disturbance is disease and it's absence is health.

---

[140] Iyengar.B.K.S., <u>YOGA, The Path to Holistic Health</u>, Dorling Kindersley, London, 2001, P.240

[141] Satyapal, Dholandass Aggarwal, <u>Yogasanas and Sadhana</u>, Pusthak Mahal, New Delhi 2003, P.47

[142] Julie Friedeberger, <u>Office Yoga</u>, Motilal Banarsidass Publishers, New Delhi, 1998, P.18.

[143] Joshi.K.S., <u>Yoga and Personality</u>, Udyana Publications, Allahabad, 1967, P.126

[144] Richmond Sonya, <u>How to be Healthy with Yoga</u>, Bell Publishing, New York, 1962, P.71

[145] Vivekananda Swamy, <u>The Complete Works of Swami Vivekananda</u>, Adwaita Ashrama, Culcutta, 1989, P.39

Nowadays Yoga is used more for therapeutic purposes.[146] Many discoveries were made at Kaivalyadhama Institute of Yoga practices, about the therapeutic effects on certain ailments.[147] At the Institute Swamy Kuvalayananda treated patients, resorting only to yogic techniques.

The nature of all yogic practices is psycho–physiological. The physiological view is that yoga helps to tone up the entire body.[148] Asanas have a profound influence on the fitness. It influences on increasing the flexiblity of the spine and the joints.[149] Yogic therapy re-establish the normal physiological functions of the body through the practice of asanas and pranayama.[150] In Yoga Therapy, the origin and development of the ailment are careully studied. The aim is not simply to cure the symptom, but to target the cause. [151]

---

[146] Saraswathy Karmananda Swamy, <u>Yogic Management of Common Diseases</u>, Bihar School of Yoga, Munger, Bihar,1968, P.19

[147] Kuvalayananda Swami, Vinekar.S.L, <u>Yoga Therapy; It's Basic Principles and Methods,</u> Central Health Education Bureau, Ministry of Health, Govt.of India, New Delhi, 1973.

[148] Hari OmGupta, <u>Yoga & Pranayama</u>, Ashirwad Sunrays, Ludhiyana, 2005, P.107

[149] Karel Werner, <u>Yoga and Indian Philosophy</u>, Motilal Banarsidass Publishers, New Delhi, 1977, P.168

[150] Jayadeva Yogendra, J.Clement Vaz, <u>The Friends of Yoga Society,</u> The Macmillan Company of India (P) Ltd, Madras, 1971, P.178

[151] Garde.R.K, <u>Principles and Practice of Yoga Therapy</u>, D.B.Taraporevala & Sons, Bombay, 1972, P.63

1.3.5 Yogic Practices and Low Back Pain

Yoga as therapy applies yogic techniques to restore health or full physical and mental functioning.[152] Yoga serves to improve, posture, flexibility, range of motion, concentration and digestion. It is a therapy for low back ache and arthritis.[153] Yoga helps to reduce the pain in lower and upper back by stretching and strengthening the different parts of the spine as well as the back bone.[154] Yoga is excellent in keeping the body limber and in shape. Pranayama and asanas reduce tension and stress that can contribute to lower back pain.[155] In Yoga, the attention is directed inward, the body receives messages that the individual is safe and secure. So muscles relax, blood pressure drops, nerves are calmed, anxiety is decreased, immunity is heightened, and healing is enhanced. These things greatly improve one's ability to deal with both the symptoms and causes of low back pain.[156]

Strengthening from Holding Yoga Positions

---

[152] George Feuerstein, Larry Payne, Yoga for Dummies, Wiley Dreamtech India (P) Ltd, New Delhi, 2006, P. 21

[153] Agrawal.S.S., Paridhavi.M., Herbal Drug Technology, Universities Press (India) Pvt. Ltd, Hyderabad, 2007, P.14

[154] Moorthy.A M., David Manual Raj.J., Yoga for Health, M.J.Publishers, Madras, 1983, P.3

[155] Sarno John, The Mind Body Connection in Yoga, Warner Books, Claton South, 1996, P.81

[156] Motiwala, Sam.N. et al, Treating Chronic Ailments with Yoga, Yoga Rahasya, 2001, 8 (2) 12-13

Postures in Yoga, strengthen the muscles in the lower back and abdomen which help the body to maintain proper upright posture and movement.[157] Yoga incorporates stretching and relaxation, which reduces tension in the lower back. Stretching the hamstring muscles helps expand the motion in the pelvis and decrease stress across the lower back.[158]

Posture, Balance and Body alignment through Yoga

Yoga poses train the body to have proper body alignment and good posture, which is an important factor in reducing low back pain.[159] Muscular fibres become strong and elastic due to the passive or active contraction and stretches in yoga. The joints get flexibility because of the manipulations and this reduces the rate of bone degeneration.[160] Couch has devised a method of teaching how to stand, sit, walk and practice yoga in "balance". He has found out that, mimicking the actions of "balanced", individuals eliminates musculo-skeletal pains and low back pain.[161] A common reason why people get into Yogic practices is for relief from low back pain and as an alternate treatment for

---

[157] Ananda Sri, The Complete Book of Yoga - Harmony of Body and Mind, Orient Paperbacks, New Delhi, 1999, P.39

[158] Sharma.P.D., Yogasana & Pranayama for Health, Navneet Publications (P) Ltd, Ahemadabad, 1984, P.117

[159] Mary Pullig Schatz, Yoga for Back Pain, Rodmell Press, Berkeley, 1992, P.87

[160] Carrmine Ireene, Yoga for Backache, Jaico publishing House, Mumbai, 2005, PP.23-24

[161] Jean Couch, The Runners' Yoga Book, Rodmell Press, Berkeley, 1991, P.86

herniated vertebral discs. [162] Keeping back in bend posture for long, causes low back ache and lumbago. Relaxation in prone position with complete breath gives relief to low back pain. [163]

Modern developments lead man to a sedentary lifestyle which results in putting on weight and weakening of the muscles for which Yoga has solution. [164] Yogasanas deal with the condition in a wholesome manner by suggesting exercises to tone and strengthen the abdomen and the lower back and removes the root cause of low back ache. [165] When the body is unable to deal with the toxins built up in the human body through a normal process of elimination, these are thrown to the joints so as to safe guard the vital organs. The joints are therefore prime sites for the build up of toxins, which cause stiffness and discomfort. Practice of Yogic exercises speed up the removal of toxins and and thereby eliminates the pain. [166] Low back pain is mainly due to the lack of exercises required for the lumbar spine, joints, back muscles and nervous

---

[162] Thomas Griner, <u>What Really Wrong with You- A Revolutionary Look at How Muscles Affect Your Health</u>, Avery Publications, New York, 1996, P.78

[163] Bhagavan Dev Acharya, <u>Yoga for Better Health</u>, Diamond Pocket Books, New Delhi, 2003, P.83

[164] Rajendra.K.V., <u>Treat Your Spinal Problem with out Drugs</u>, Institute of Naturopathy & Yogic Sciences, Jindal Nagar, Bangalore, 1997, P.63

[165] Nisha Varma, <u>YOGA for Back Problems</u>, Brijbasi Art Press & Publishers, Noida, 2006, P.76

[166] Sunny Chennat (Yoga Master), Yoga & Disease Cure, Coral Books, Kottayam, 2004, P.62.

system. Selected yogasanas are very helpful in eliminating low back pain without the application any drugs.[167] Yoga helps people concentrate their energy on breathing and maintaining posture. This action coupled with the poses is said to dissipate stress and anxiety, therefore, relieving pain in the lower back.[168]

1.4 NATUROPATHY

Naturopathy [168 A] is defined as a way of treating illness which works on the priniciple that healing depends upon the action of natural healing forces, present in the human body. The concept of "vis medicatrix naturae"; the healing power of the nature, is very ancient. It was Hippocrates who first, realized the importance of nature's own healing powers. To him disease is an effort of the body to establish the disturbed equilibrium of the body function.

Naturopathy is the natural method, which far excels the other systems, is the foundation of the new art of healing without drugs or operation.[169] Naturopathy is the science which deals with the correction of bodily disorders

---

[167] Chidhambaran.T.G. (Yogacharya), <u>Yoga, A Style of Life,</u> Amulya Publications, Kochi, 1985, PP.337-338.

[168] Nagrathana.R, & Narendra.R., <u>Yoga for Common Ailments,</u> Gaia Books, London, 1990

[168 A] Andrew Stanway, <u>Alternate Medicine (A guide to Natural Therapies),</u> Chancellor Press, London, 1986, P.104

[169] Louis Kuhne, <u>Neo-Naturopathy, The New Science of Healing,</u> Kitabistan, Allahabad, 1967, P.12

and restoration of health through elements available in nature. [170] Naturopathy aims to diagnose and treat any human disease, pain, injury and deformity by the use of air,light, water, heat and such other natural means.[171] According to Neuberger, author of "The Doctrine of the healing powers of nature through the course of Time", "Nature is the healer of diseases". [172] The science of natural therapeutics is based on the use of five elements which constitute the human body; ie earth, water, ether, sunlight and air.[173] Naturopathy [174] is based on the principle of co-operation with the natural laws of life which are for ever working within the human body. Naturopathy works on the principle that acute disease is simply a manifestation of the healing forces' effort to get the body back to normal.[175] Naturopathy relies upon the use of Herbs, food grown without artificial fertilizers, pure water, sun light and fresh air in an effort to rid the body

---

[170] Bolar.P.K., Foreword to A Complete Hand book of Nature Cure by H.K.Bakhru, Jaico Publishing House, Bombay, 1991, P.3

[171] Jussawalla.J.M., The Key to Nature Cure, Sangam Books Ltd, London, 1992, P.2

[172] Sreenivasan.H., Nature Cure – Origin and Development of the Fundamental Principles, National Book Stall, Kottayam, Kerala, 1996, P.18

[173] Gandhi.M.K., Key to Health, Navjivan Publishing House, Ahmedabad, 1948, P.30

[174] Singh.S.J., History and Philosophy of Naturopathy, Nature cure Research Hospital, Lucknow, 1980, P.25

[175] Rajkumar Pruthi, Hand Book of Alternative Therapies, UBS Publishers' Distributors (P) Ltd, New Delhi, 2004, P. 57

of "unnatural" substances,which are said to be at the root of all most all diseases.[176]

1.4.1 Natural Healing Power

Hippocrates said; " Let your Food be your Medicine and your Medicine be your Food ".[177] This clearly indicates what nature cure is. Nature cure is a philosophy of disease and healing, which resorts to nothing but the simplest and most natural measures to bring about results.[178] Nature cure is a system of man building in harmony with the constructive principle in nature on the physical, mental and moral planes of being.[179] A man who accepts nature cure, takes steps to cure himself by eliminating poisons from the system and takes precautions against falling ill in the future.[180] In Nature cure no poisonous or intoxicating medicine is administered. it is the way of leading real life, which if adopted, none will ever be ill. Along with simple living, it eliminates or rather uproots the

---

[176] Harrison.L.M., The Pocket Medical Dictionay, CBS Publishers, New Delhi, 1986, P.273

[177] Vaughan.JG, Judd.PA, The Oxford Book of Health Foods, Oxford University Press Inc, New York, 2003, (in Preface)

[178] Harry Benjamin , Everybody's Guide to Nature Cure, Health for all Publishing Company, Great Britain, 1952, P.9

[179] Henry Lindlahr, Philosophy and Practice of Nature Cure, Satysahitya Sahyogi Sangh, Hyderabad, 1986, P.22

[180] Gandhi.M.K., NATURE CURE (edited by Bharathan Kumarappa), Navjeevan Publishing House, Ahemmedabad, 1954, P.44

diseases.[181] Nature cure is based on the realization that Human Beings are born healthy and strong and that he/ she can stay as such, by living in accordance with the laws of nature.[182] All forms of diseases are due to the same cause; the accumilation of waste materials in the system. All acute diseases are nothing more than self-initiated efforts by the body to throw off the accumilated waste materials and all chronic diseases are the results of the continued suppression of the acute diseases through harmful methods such as drugs, vaccines etc. The body contains an elaborate healing mechanism, which has a power to bring about a return to normal health, provided right methods are employed to enable it to do.[183] Nature cure treatment is the sum total of activities directed towards helping a patient. The focus is to relieve the immediate physical pain and at large to modify his behaviour patterns which may give him positive results.[184] Dr.Koner opined,[185] "Nature's healing force, makes steady progress, forwards recovery in all diseases, if the patient acts according to Naturopathic treatment" .Over the centuries, man has discovered that in case he falls a victim to disease

---

[181] Gouri Shankar, <u>Publishers Note in Scientific Nature Cure by Dr.Hira Lal</u>, Gandhi Smarak Prakrithik Chikitsa Parishad, New Delhi, 1993, P.V

[182] Jussawalla.J.M., <u>Prevention is Better than Cure</u>, Jaico Publishing House, Bombay, 1961, P.28

[183] Bakhru.H.K., <u>A complete Hand book of Nature Cure</u>, Jaico Publishing House, Mumbai 1991, PP 4-5.

[184] Misra.P.D., Beena Misra, <u>Nature Cure-Philosophy and Methods</u>, B.I.Churchill Livingstone Pvt.Ltd, New Delhi , 1998, P.93

[185] Kulkarni.V.M., <u>Naturopathy, Art of Drugless Healing</u>, Sri Satguru Publications, New Delhi, 1986, P.26

due to unavoidable causes, he can recoup his health quickly by utilizing "Nature" to cure the illness speedly and successfully. [186]

Diseases are the manifestation of the violation of the "natural laws". The unnatural way of food habits and life style causes severe damage to the vital force of the individual, which is the main reason for various diseases.[187] Nature cure means all methods of treating diseases which aim at cooperating with the natural forces and defensive mechanism of the body.[188] Nature cure and Yoga are complimentary to each other. In a broader sense, yoga is a part of nature cure as it also promotes healthy functioning of both body and mind.[189] Ellis Barker said, "very likely the whole fundamental concept, that the micro organisms create the diseases, on which modern bacteriology has been errected, is utterly and preposterously wrong, for it may be that in absolute opposition to this concept, the disease creates the micro organism.[190] Mahatma Gandhi was very much impressed with the curing methods of Naturopathy and he himself experimented with the treatment with water, sun light and mud, and found as

---

[186] Vethathiri Maharishi Yogiraj, <u>Simplified Physical Exercises,</u> Vethathiri Publications, Erode, Tamil Nadu, 2002, P.7

[187] Kayyoleth.D.K., <u>Complete Naturopathy,</u> Pen Books, Aluva, Kochi, 2006, P.155

[188] Jussawalla.J.M., <u>Healing from Within</u>, Manaktalas Publishers, Bombay, 1996, P. 6.

[189] Xavier Cherupallikkatt, <u>Nature Cure</u>, Deepika Book House Kottayam, Kerala, 1979, P.48

[190] Gala.D.R., Dhiren Gala, Sanjay Gala, <u>Nature Cure for Common Diseases</u>, Navneeth Publications (India) Ltd, Mumbai, 1998, P.17

very effective in reducing various ailments. [191] "We are not treating illness" says naturopaths."We are inducing health". It is much more positive.[192] Nature cure believes that human body has the spores of germs that grow and multiply only in morbid matter. Therefore, it's prescripion is to purify the body regularly to prevent the growth of germs, in order to develop immunity.[193] Naturopatnic treatment include nutritional food and therapeutic fasting; herbs, minerals, and vitamins; counselling, massage, colonic enemas; hydrotherapy, heat, and cold applications; therapeutic exercise etc.[194] According to Gandhiji,[195] all most all diseases could be cured by means of well regulated diet, water and earth treatment and similar naturopathic remedies.

1.4.2 Role of Food in Naturopathy.

Natural foods have "Life Force" ie; their enzymes. Enzymes have magnetic, cosmic energy which activates substances. It is a form of "prana"- the life energy which, controls almost all the body processes of human beings.[196]

---

[191] Rajeswari.P, <u>Nature Cure at Home</u>, Kwality Printing & Publishing Company, New Delhi, 1998, P.14

[192] Nilamboor.K.R.C (Dr.), <u>Yoga, Food – Nature's Medicine</u>, Poorna Publications, Kozhikode, 2003, P.43

[193] Henry Lindlahr, <u>Practice of Natural Therapeutics</u>, Sat Sahitya Sahyogi Sangh, Hyderabad, 1990, P 9

[194] Jacobs.J.W., <u>Complimentary/Alternative Medicine, An evidence based approach</u>, Mosby INC, St Louis, 1999, P.27

[195] Gandhi.M.K., <u>The Story of My Experiments with Truth</u>, Navjivan Publishing House, Ahmedabad, 1929, P.226

Wigmore says; "guided by spiritual mentality and nourished only by live uncooked food, the human body will run indefinitely, unhampered by sickness.[197]

Food is defined as those thing which gives energy and nourishment to the body. Sunlight, water, air and fasting/rest provides enough energy to the body and hence these can be said to be as Food. This is the basis of Naturopathy.[198] Food affects every organ of human body and the correct diet encourage fitness and enegy, nourishes the nerves, feed muscles, improve blood circulation and breathing and support the immune system.[199] No food that is cooked can possibly called a natural food. It is possible for anyone to live in good health on nothing, but a small amount of fruits, vegetables and nuts as these are in natural form.[200] The food we eat, is like fuel. It gives the body the energy it need to function well. Healthy food is the key to well being.[201] Food is the chief source of essential nutrients which the body needs for it's well being. Good food is

---

[196] Dewan.A.P., <u>Food For Health,</u> A.C.Specialist Publishers (P) Ltd, New Delhi, 1996, (Preface).

[197] Ann Wigmore, <u>Be Your Own Doctor,</u> Hemisphere Press Inc, New York, 1988, P.5

[198] Thomas Malieckal, <u>Food is Medicine,</u> Nature Cure Hospital, Moozhikkulam, Kerala 1997, P.38

[199] Geddes, Grosset, <u>Guide to Natural Healing,</u> Davi Dale House, New Lanark, Scotland 1997, P.261

[200] William.H.Hay., <u>Health and Foods,</u> Sree Niwas Publications, Jaipur, 2005, P.152.

[201] Gillian McKeith, <u>You are what You Eat,</u> Penguin Books, New Delhi, 2004, P.13

indispensable for health in all stages of life.[202] It has long been recognized that adequate nutrition is necessary for good health, immunity and optimal efficiency.[203] The human body is not designed to digest more than one concentrated food (which is not a fruit or vegetable). Food combining is based on the theory that certain combinations of food may be digested with greater ease.[204] Doctors all over the world have hailed the exciting discovery that food can cure and heal. Now they have realized the curative powers of food.[205]

It is accepted that most of the diseases are caused by wrong food. It is through bad digestion that foreign matter is formed in the body and thus diseases develop. For the proper flow of "prana" (vital power), the right food is a must.[206] Hira Lal, has mentioned the following rules for eating.[207] The daily meals should include fruits and raw green vegetables. Two or three compatible foods should be taken together. Must eat only when the body demands food. It is advisable to eat fresh natural foods (which do not contain any additives or synthetic

---

[202] Kusum Gupta, <u>Food and Nutrition – Facts and Figures</u>, Jaypee Brothers (Medical Publishers), New Delhi, 1986 (Preface to the first edn.)

[203] Herbert Pallack, Seymour.L.Halpern, <u>Nutritional Data</u> (3rd edn), H.J.HEINZ Company, Pennsylvania, 1956, P.86

[204] Harvey Marilyn Diamond, <u>Fit For Life</u>, Bentham Books, London, 1987, P.148.

[205] Thanu Shree Podder, <u>The Ultimate food for Body, Mind and Soul</u>, UBS Publishers & Distributors Pvt Ltd, New Delhi, 2006, P.92

[206] Louis Kuhne, <u>The New Science of Healing</u>, Kitabistan, Allahabad, 1967, P.79

[207] Hira Lal, <u>Scientific Nature Cure</u>, Gandhi Smarak Prakratik Chikitsa Parishad, New Delhi, 1993, P 83

ingradients)   for maintaining proper health.[208] The food we eat form the foundation of every cell in the body and when they are the right foods, they contribute to the right tissues, organs, muscles and bones. Here the energy level will be high and the body becomes stronger.[209] Ramana Maharshi said; "Eat without thinking of the ego, then what you eat becomes God's Blessing."[210] Improper bowels are the main reason for most of the diseases and the reason behind is the consumption of improper food. Natural foods helps bowels to move properly and avoids the possibility of many diseases.[211] In an ideal food, it is essential to ensure enough of proteins, fats and carbohydrates to facilitate an active life. Minerals, water and vitamins are also needed to break down these and convert them into energy, must be included in the diet.[212]

It is immaterial whether we eat nourishing food or not, but the question is how much of it, is assimilated by the body. There must be sufficient intervals between the off-take of food.[213] The vitamins contained in the food play a vital

---

[208] Shubhangini.A.Joshi., <u>Nutrition and Dietitics,</u> Tata McGraw-Hill Publishers, New Delhi, 2002, P.11

[209] Phoebe Phillips, Pamela Hatch, <u>The Best of Good Health</u>, Unwin Paperbacks, London, 1978, P.46

[210] VenkitaRam.T.N., <u>Maharshi's Gospel, Book i and ii,</u> Sri Ramanasramam,Thirunelveli, 1994, P.36

[211] Dileep Kulkarni, <u>Ahead to Nature</u>, Vivekananda Kendra Publication Trust, Chennai, 1998, P.153

[212] Rajeev Sharma, <u>A Complete Guide of Naturopathy</u>, Indiana Publishing House, New Delhi 2006, P.562

role in influencing the endocrine glands which produces hormones. When vegetables are cooked, the vitamins burnt away and destroyed by fire and thus human body won't get the real benefit from the food. Hence vegetables should be eaten as 'raw'.[214] By cooking and frying the food stuff, the inorganic salts of calcium, ferrum, pottassium, magnesium, sodium, phosphorus, sulphur, iodine, bromine etc is lost. Without these our body will not develop properly.[215] Good blood circulation and elimination of uric acid are important factors in staying free of aches and pains. Increase the off take of food that are rich in minerals, foods that promotes detoxification and foods that are diuretic. Calcium and vitamin D help to strengthen the bones.[216]

Water helps to flush out the excess acid particularly from the kidneys. Eat more green leafy vegetables and nuts such as Walnut and Almonds. Add more raw fruits and raw vegetables into the daily food.[217] The vegetarian diet contains the "real natural food", which is high in fibre and starchy carbohydrates. Nuts and beans are protein rich foods. Dried fruits provide iron, cereals provide

---

[213]   Raghavan Thirumulppad.K., <u>Prakriti Chikitsa (Nature Cure)</u>, Alter Media & Grass Hopper Publishers, Trichur, Kerala, 1957, P.22

[214]   Kulkarni.V.M., <u>Naturopathy, the Art of Drugless Healing</u>, Sri Satguru Publications, New Delhi, 1986, P.247

[215]   Carlson Wade, <u>Health Secrets from the Orient</u>, Allied Publishers (Pvt) Ltd, New Delhi, 1997, P.179

[216]   Pierre Jean Cousin, <u>Food is Medicine</u>, Duncan Baird Publishers, London, 2001, P.60

[217] Gillian McKeith, <u>You are what You Eat</u>, Penguin Books, New Delhi, 2004, PP.140-141

vitamin B and fresh fruits provide Vitamin C.[218] Bone and cartilage strengthening vitamins such as Vitamin C & Vitamin D and minerals such as calcium, magnesium and manganese which are essential for bone strengthening are obtained from naturopathic way of food habits.[219] Most of the diseases are amenable through Food therapy. "Food is the best medicine." This is the main slogan of Nature Cure.[220] Nutrition and Dietitics in Naturopathy includes the prescription of a balanced wholesome, natural diet.[221] The controlled abstinence from food (Fasting) has been used therapeutically for over 2,000 years. It allows the body to concentrate its resources on dealing with the disease rather than the processes of digestion.[222]

No one aspect is more important than another. What is eaten, for example, is dependent on how it is eaten and when, in what frame of mind and in what physical condition of the individual.[223] Georgiou says; "It is advisable for the patients to under go a detoxification diet with fruits and vegetables for 15 days, which helps to bring the body back to its normal alkaline state because an acidic

---

[218] Liz Burnell, Nicola Mcclure, Michael.J.Sadler, <u>Eating Well,</u> World Bank INC, Chicago, 1993, P.44

[219] Anand Raj Mool, <u>Food for Health,</u> Sarva Seva Sangh Prakashan, Varanasi, 1989. P.29

[220] Varma.C.R.R., <u>Naturopathy,</u> Institute of Naturopathic Research, Trivandrum, 1996, P. 59

[221] Aman.Dr., <u>Medicinal Secrets of Your Food</u>, Indo American Hospital, Mysore, 1985, P.188

[222] Jayakumar.K.R., <u>Fasting,</u> D.C.Books, Kottayam, Kerala, 2003, P.51

[223] Jussawalla.J.M., <u>The Natural Way of Living,</u> Vikas Publishing House Pvt Ltd, New Delhi, 1974, P.59

body is one with far more inflammation".[224] It is better to avoid sugar, white flour, white rice, sweets, chocolate, and limit coffee consumption. Also avoid saturated and trans-fat since these can trigger inflammatory chemicals in the body.[225] Bromelain, the enzyme found in pineapple helps reduce inflammation and pain from trauma, sports injuries arthritis and back pain.[226]

Naturopathy always emphasizes much, on the use of "Good Food". There are varieties of food which are advisable for human beings and there are other varieties which are not advisable for intake by human beings.[227] The Body makes use of nourishing food whereas it tries to reject any hazardous substances, taken in to the body in the form of food.[228] The core modalities supporting the principle of naturopathy include diet modification and nutritional supplements.[229] Fresh and dry Fruits are the natural staple food for human beings. The ailments caused by the intake of unnatural foods could be treated by

---

[224] Lindlahr, Henry.M.D., Philosophy and Practice of Nature Cure, Sat Sahitya Sahyogi Sangh, Hyderabad,1988, P.41

[225] Garg.B.D.(compiled), Nature Cure Treatment, Institute of Naturopathy and Yogic Sciences, Bangalore, 1997, P.112

[226] Varghese.K.C., History of Nature Cure, Mahatma Nature Cure Centre, Thalipparamba, Kannur, 1998, P.69

[227] Mukherji.K.R., Protective Foods In Health and Diseases, Prakrithi Ckikitsalaya Publishers, Culcutta, 1983, P.83

[228] Lekshmana Sharma.K., Swaminathan.S., Speaking of Nature Cure, Sterling Publishers (Pvt) Ltd, New Delhi, 1995, P.59

[229] Singh.S.J., Food Remedies, Nature Cure Council of Medical Research, Lucknow, 1982, P.126

fresh and dry fruits since these are not only good food but also a good medicine.[230] To attain good health, it is essential to follow the rules of good nutrition and regular exercise. A nutritious diet, proper lifestyle, adequate sleep and exercise are instrumental in keeping the human body free of all ailments.[231] If the individual wants to be vibrantly and vigorously alive, he/she has to eat food that's alive. Fruits have the highest energy of all foods.[232]

Juicy fruits, tubers, legumes, ripe fruits, leafy and root vegetables which are alkaline-forming, should constitute 80% of our daily diet. The other 20% of the diet should consists of acid-forming food containing concentrated protein and starches like nuts, dates, cereals etc.[233] The "Grape Cure" is perhaps the best of the various fruit cures proposed from time to time and a remedy for various diesases.[234] Lemon is useful for curing sciatica, Lumbago etc. Lemon is used as a medicine in Naturopathy as it alkalises the blood.[235] Orange being an excellent source of Calcium and Vitamin C, is valuable in the diseases of the bones.

---

[230] Bakhru.H.K., <u>Foods that Heal – The Natural Way to Good Health</u>, Orient Paper Backs, New Delhi, 1990, P.13

[231] Harry Benjamin, <u>Our Diet in Heath and Diseases</u>, Wilco Publishing House, Bombay, 1991, P.80

[232] Edison.K., <u>Fruits and Treatment</u>, Mayoora Publications, Trivandrum, 2001, P.29

[233] Rajendra.K.V., Jinda.S.R., Rehman.A.., <u>Treat Your Spinal problem without Drugs</u>, Institute of Naturopathy and Yogic Science, Bangalore, 1997, PP.32-33

[234] Johanya Brandt, <u>The Grape Cure</u>, Ehret Literature Publishing Co, California, 1998, P.147

[235] Govindan Nair (Yogacharya), <u>Health and Longevity</u>, D.C.Books, Kottayam, 2001, P.103

Vitamin C protects the synovial membranes.[236] The beneficial aspect of fruits is essentially in their vitamins, minerals and enzyme contents. They defend the body against so called "free radicals", which are molecules that damage the cells. [237]

It is believed that all living beings are a composite of the five basic elements ie; Earth, Water, Fire, Air and Sky. In order to keep life going, it is important to replenish these elements through natural foods.[238] Juice of fruits and vegetables is more preferable as it takes far less time to digest and thus speed up the absorption of vitamins and minerals by the body.[239] Juice of vegetables or their use in raw form should be an essential part of one's routine dietary menu. Vegetable juice not only corrects defective metabolism but is also capable of repairing torn and worn out tissues.[240]

1.4.3 Role of Herbs in Naturopathy

Every culture has a rich herbal lore and broad repertoire of remedies for conditions that commonly affect it's people. This they have achieved by means

---

[236] Braverman.J.B.S., <u>Citrous Fruits</u>, Interscience Publishers Inc, New York, 1949, P.31

[237] Ganapathy Singh Verma.K.V.J., <u>Miracles of Fruits,</u> The Rasayan Pharmacy, New Delhi, 1978, P.29

[238] Balakrishnan.V.V., <u>Fruits & Vegetables and their Medicinal Properties</u>, D.C.Books, Kottayam, 1988, P.62

[239] Susane.E.Charmine, <u>The Complete Raw Juice Therapy</u>, Thorsons Publishing Group, London, 1987, P.49

[240] Walter.N.F., <u>Raw Vegetable Juices</u>, Jove Books, New York, 1983, P.57

of Herbal Therapy.[241] It was impossible to cure any diseases in the past without the use of herbs, when the human beings were ignorant of other alternative treatments.[242] The chemical compounds in herbs have through time and experience, come tobe considered the active agents – stimulants, inhibitors, supplements or synthesizers. The second aspect of herb medicine is that of energies.[243] In nature cure, use of herbs has a significant role, both as an agent for healing and for improving general health. [244]

1.4.4 Naturopathy and Low back pain

Human body has a natural ability to heal itself and to fight infection and to repair the damaged tissues. So it could be the same with the low back of human beings. Certainly the lower back also is able to heal itself.[245] Degenerative disorders resulting in spinal problems (eg. low back ache) are not merely mechanical problems. According to "Natural Dietetics", the point to be considered is the inability of the digestive process to supply calcium and other minerals to the bone structures, even when the person is consuming mineral rich

---

[241] Aviva Jill Roman, <u>Natural Healing</u>, Sree Satguru Publishers, New Delhi, 1996, P.14

[242] Dartur.J.F., <u>Medicinal Plants of India</u> , D.B.Taraporevala Sons & Co, Bombay, 1985, P.13

[243] Humbart Santillo, <u>Natural Healing with Herbs</u>, Crest Publishing House, New Delhi, 2001, P.xviii

[244] Joseph Chittoor (Fr.), Purushothaman.C.K., <u>Herbals and Treatment of Diseases</u>, Samskruthi Publications, Kannur, 1993, P.124

[245] Sunitha Pant Bansal, <u>Healing Power of Foods</u>, Pusthak Mahal , New Delhi, 2006,P.82

food.[246] Naturopathic diet and simple exercises can do a lot in the "self healing process" of the human body. Naturopathy treatment can be effective enough to cure the arthritis pain and lower back pain.[247] When a bone is broken, the intelligent power that built our body immedaitely sets to repair the damaged bone by the same process of cell metabolism, we saw in healing of the wound, the fracture parts are reunited.[248]

1.4.5 Naturopathic Method of Treatment

The common naturopathic methods of treatment[249] include correct dieting to rebuild the tissues, graduated exercises used to correct structural defects and encourage drainage and circulation, Deep breathing of fresh air, sufficient physiological rest, varieties of hydropathic treatment. As the patient takes to the nature cure programme of dieting etc, the vital powers in him engage itself in rebuilding of the damaged tissues from within.[250] In order to treat low Backache

---

[246] Hira Lal.M, <u>Scientific Nature Cure</u>, Gandhi Smaraka Nature Cure Parishad, New Delhi, 1987, P.128

[247] Modi.P.L, Vithaldas.K, <u>Nature Cure for Common Diseases</u>, Orient Paper Backs, New Delhi, 1982, P.92

[248] Singh.S.J.,<u>History</u> and Philosophy of Naturopathy, Nature Cure Prints & Publishers, Lucknow, 1980, P.533

[249] Kunhe Louis, <u>Neo Naturopathy – The New Science of Healing</u>, Kitabistan, Allahabad, 1967, P.93

[250] Lekshmana Sharma.K., <u>Practical Nature Cure</u>, The Nature Cure Publishing House, Puthukottai, Tamil Nadu, 1990, P.575

naturally, the following things have to done.[251] Take only the natural diet and flush the bowels out weekly with enema. Discontinue the use of meat, coffee, tea and other kidney damaging foods.

1.4.6 Baths as remedy for low back pain

Kneipp[252] has discovered that the cold water bath is capable of curing Sciatica. Water application consisted of a complete lavation (every night), an upper affusion (Fore noon), a back affussion (after noon), a semi bath (every second day), Knee affusion, was found to be effective against Sciatica. Water was considered as an important element of the cure of so many diseases. The waters (are) indeed medicinal, the waters (are) the "amiva dispellers" (and) the waters (are) medicines for every (diseases). Therefore let them (be) medicines for you.[253] Warm and Hot Bath soothe the cutanious nerves and nerves of internal organs. Hot Bath stimulates the nerves and also relieves pain including in the lower back.[254]

Hip Bath and Spinal Bath, invented by Louis Kuhne, are very effective in reducing pain at the lower back. In both these baths, blood circulation increases

---

[251] Ganapathy Singh Verma.K.V.J., <u>Miracles of Indian Herbs,</u> The Rasayan Pharmacy, New Delhi, 1982, P.46

[252] Sebastian Kneipp, <u>My Water-Cure,</u> Pilgrims Books (P) Ltd, New Delhi, 1998, P.243

[253] Kenneth.G.Zysk, <u>Medicine in the Veda (Religious Healing in the Veda),</u> Motilal Banarsidass Publishers, New Delhi, 1996, P.90

[254] Singh.S.J., <u>BATHS-The Treatment of Diseases By the Use of Water, Light, Mud, Vapour and Air,</u> Nature Cure Research Hospital, Lucknow, 1963, P.30

to the lower back which in turn reduces muscle spasm and relieves the pain.[255] The patient may take the spinal bath daily. Use the non violent enema as and when necessary and live hygenically, paying attention to the priciples of vital energy. This will ultimately helps to reduce the pain in the lower back.[256]

Sun Bath may be done when the sun has risen some what high in the sky and it's heat is mild. The patient may begin with 5 minutes and gradually increase it up to 20 minutes. Sun bath is so beneficial to osteoporotic patients.[257] Sun light is used in Naturopathy for joint problems and back pain. It is a natural source of Vitamin D and is inevitable for strengthening the bones.[258] Vitamin D helps calcium and Phosphorus to build bones. Sun light is a good source of Vitamin D.[259] In Mud bath, dried mud obtained from volcanic regions, which contains mineral matter is used for the relief of pain.[260]

---

[255] Kulkarni.V.M., <u>Drugless Prevention and Cure of Disease with Water</u>, Crest Publishing House, New Delhi, 1997, P.118

[256] Somanath.K.B. (Translated from Herbert.M.Shelton), <u>A Preface to the Drugless Therapy</u>, Prakruthi Publications, Thrissur, 1991, P.28

[257] Dayanandan.P., <u>Nature Cure for Health and Logivity</u>, Jihwa Publications, Kottayam, Kerala, 2005, P.73

[258] Charu.V.Bhatnagar, <u>Naturopathy</u>, Dapu Nature Cure Hospital Journal, Nature Cure and Yoga Trust, New Delhi , October 1992, P.16

[259] Chalkley.A.M., <u>A Text book for the Health Worker</u>, New Age International (P) Ltd Publishers, New Delhi, 2005, P.214

[260] Jayamoni.C.V., <u>Health Management – A New Perspective</u>, Institute of Naturopathic Research, Trivandrum, 1999, P.59

Massage is beneficial for back aches in Naturopathy. In Naturopathic massage, Rose Mary, Petitgrain and Lavender are used to reduce the pain.[261] In Friction massage, circular massage is done over and around the joints and the painful areas. It helps to tone up the muscles and the tendons of the joints. It reduces the pain and swelling due to inflammation.[262] Mustard Oil massage is found to be effective in reducing the pain caused by Sciatica.[263] Philipose says; Massage and non violent enema as means of nature cure, are beneficial for the relief of low back pain.[264]

According to Sharma; 15 minutes of Hydro Massage, 11 minutes of Hot and cold jet Spray and 17 minutes of Hot and cold spinal bath relieve Low Back Pain.[265] Raghavan[266] says that, instead of treating symptoms, Naturopathy seeks to identify and treat the underlying causes. Naturopathy is particularly well suited for chronic conditions such as muscular pain, Arthritis, Back ache etc.

---

[261] Cathy Hopkins, Thorsons Principles of Aromatherapy, Harper Collins Publishers, London, 1996, P.141

[262] Devaraj.T.L., Nature Cure for Common Diseases, Lotus Press, New Delhi, 1998, P.24

[263] Ibrahim.K.K., Health at the Finger Tips, Current Books, Trichur, Kerala, 2007, P.167

[264] Philipose.P.A.Pullippadavil, Nature Cure – Diseases and Remedies, Maria Publishers, Palghat, Kerala, 1993, P.64

[265] Rajeev Sharma, A Non-Harming Therapy – NATUROPATHY, Manoj Publications, New Delhi, 2004, P.146

[266] Raghavan.D., Nature Cure and Allopathy – A Comparative Study, Prakarthi Chikitsa Pracharaka Samithi, Kannur, Kerala, 1997, P.71

Nature cure is a method of treating various diseases using food, exercises and heat to assist the natural healing process of the body. [267] John Powathil [268] says; Naturopathy believes that all forms of diseases are due to the same cause; the accumilation of toxins in human body. Nature cure also believes that "disease is one, it's cause is one and so it's treatment is one".

According to Clark,[269] for low back ache, the most important supplement is magnesium to cleanse the kidneys. Minerals like calcium and magnesium relax the muscles which provide pain relief. The splendour of the Naturopathic approach is that each individual is treated as unique. The same is the case of low back pain too.[270]

1.5 PHYSIOTHERAPY

Physiotherapy is a health care programme concerned with human function and movement and maximising potential. It uses physical approaches to promote, maintain and restore physical, psychological and social well being, taking account of variations in health status. The exercise of clinical judgement and informed interpretations is at it's core.[271]

---

[267] Subhash.K., <u>Modern Nature Cure</u>, Kalpadrumam Publications, Trivandrum, 1999, P.129

[268] John Powathil, <u>Man , Health and Diseases,</u> Pen Books (P) Ltd, Aluva, Kerala, 2006, P.62

[269] Linda Clark, <u>Hand Book of Natural Remedies for Common Ailments</u>, Pocket Books, New York, 1976, P.45

[270] Wendy Gist, <u>Low Back Pain: A Naturopathic Approach,</u> Positive Health Magazine, Issue 138, August 2007

The role of physiotherapy is to minimize the difference between a person's current movement capability and his or her preferred movement capability.[272] The Physical agents that are used for the application of external energy to achieve the therapeutic effects in human body include Heat, Ultra sound, Infra red rays, Massage, Electrical nerve stimulator, Interferential current therapy and Short Wave Diathermy.[273] The role of the physiotherapist is to provide education and advice to the patient in physical activities such as lifting and carring. The physiotherapist uses Heat, Cold, Massage, Traction, Exercises, Mobilization, Manipulation, Analgesics, Anti-inflammatory drugs, Injections etc to eliminate the pain.[273 A]

Rankin[274] says that exercise therapy may help chronic low back pain patients, return to normal daily activities. Education, active exercise programmes and relaxation exercises can improve long-term outcomes for pain and functional status compared with other treatments for chronic low back pain. The major conditions managed by physiotherapists can be broadly grouped into three

---

[271] Chartered Society of Physiotherapy, <u>Curriculam Framework for Qualifying Programmes in Physiotherapy</u>, London., 2002, P. 16

[272] Cott.C.A., Finch.E., Gasner.D., Movement Continuum theory of Physical Therapy, <u>Physiother Can</u>, 1995, 47 (2): 87-95

[273] Natarajan.R, <u>Text Book of Orthopaedics and Traumatology</u>, M.N.Orthopaedic Hospital Publishers, Madras,1991, P.163

[273 A] Jayson..M.I.V., <u>Looking After Your Back</u>, Jaico Publishing House, Bombay, 1990, P.32

[274] Gabrielle Rankin , <u>Physiotherapy,</u> Vol.91:Issue 1, March 2005, P.12

categories:[275] musculoskedletal, cardiopulmonary and neurological, out of which in Musculoskeletal physiotherapy, comes various therapeutic physiotherapy modalities such as exercise prescription (strength, motor control, stretching and endurance), manual techniques, soft tissue massage, and various forms of so-called "electrophysical agents" (such as heat therapy and electrotherapy).

Role of Physiotherapist and patient in managing Low Back Pain

Careful supervision of the patient by the physiotherapist, in concert with reinforcement from the physician, can prepare the patient to apply heat, cold, or a variety of treatments. Although the patient is given the responsibility for this part of his care, periodic follow-up and re-assessment should be done to determine changes in his physiological, psychological, and functional status.[276] Monika and Alarcos say,[277] Disability or limitations in human functioning are universal experiences that concern all people. Physical therapy aims to improve functioning and prevent disability of the individuals.For Physiotherapy, the roots of the profession can be found in massage. Physiotherapists continue to use massage therapeutically in addition to a range of other manual techniques.[278]

---

[275] Jayanth Joshi, Prakash Kotwal, Essentials of Orthopaedics and Applied Physiotherapy, B.I. Churchill Livingstone, New Delhi, 2000, P. 429

[276] Moncur.C, Shields. M.N., Baillieres Clinical Rheumatology. 1987 Apr;1(1):183-93

[277] Monica.E.Finger, Alarcos Cieza, Physical Therapy, Vol.86, No.9, Sept.2006, P.1203

[278] Stuart .B. Porter, Tidy's Physiotherapy, Reed Elsevier India Pvt Ltd, New Delhi, 2003, P.3

1.5.1 Posture

Hewes says,[279] that human beings sit, kneel, stand and recline in ways that are socially determined. It is now established that human posture, physique, and body image as well as emotions and thought patterns are culturally shaped. "Yogabhashya" says; the posture becomes perfect, when the effort of achieving it vanishes. Posture means carriage or the manner of holding one's body. So a person's good posture means, how he carries himself.[280]

There are many concepts of human posture and many interpretations of it's importance. Posture is an instrument of mechnaical efficiency, of muscle balance and of neuromuscular cordination.[281] Tense and weak muscles induced by poor posture can cause restricted owkward and painful movements. The harmonious muscle functioning that follows a programme of stregthening makes painless and dynamic movement possible.[282] Good posture is the position of the body held without any sense of effort. Here the body weight is equally distributed over both the legs so as to produce least fatigue.[283]

---

[279] George Leonard, Michael Murphy; The Life We are Given, J.P.Tarcher/ Putnam Books, New York, 1995, P.188

[280] Saroj Kanta Behari, Prasanna Kumar Choudhury; Book on Health and Physical Education, Kalyani Publishers, New Delhi, 1996, P.43

[281] Moorthy.A.M., Sports Physiotherapy, Jayavel Printers and Publishers, Kottaiyur, Tamil.Nadu, 2001, P.103

[282] Pilates Patricia Lamond, Harmonious Body Control, New Holland Publishers, London 2002, P.11

[283] Benny.K.M, Health and Physical Education, V.Publishers, Kottayam, Kerala, 2006, P.244

Maintaining A Healthy Spine - Posture

Researches suggest that many spine problems including lower back ache result from poor posture and body mechanics, which subject the spine to abnormal stress.[284] Abnormal stress over time can lead to structural changes in the spine, including degeneration of disks and joints. All of these structural changes can lead to pain. A "wall test" [285] can be performed to help practice good standing posture. Stand with head, shoulders, and back against wall and heels about 5-6 inches forward. Draw in the lower abdominals, decreasing the arch in the low back. Push away from the wall and try to maintain this upright, vertical alignment.

1.5.2 Physiotherapy and Low Back Pain

David and Dennis [286] say; Rest, Analgesics, Heat, Gradual Mobilization, Lumbosacral Brace and Manipulation form the standard treatment for low back pain. According to Maheswari,[287] Use of heat therapy (hot pack, Short-wave diathermy, ultra sound etc) and spine exercise programme are much beneficial

---

[284] Gonzalez.E.G.,Materson.R.S., The Management of Acute Low Back Pain, Demos Vermande, New York, 1997, P.91

[285] Donald Norfolk, Conquering Back Pain, Blandford Press, London, 1997, PP.32-34

[286] David.J.Dandy, Dennis.J.Edwards; Essentials of Orthopaedics and Trauma, Churchill Livingstone, Edinburgh, 2001, P.425

[287] Maheswari.J., Essential Orthopaedics, Mehtha Publishers, New Delhi, 1993, P 241.

for treating low back pain. It is advisable to use corset as a temporary measure in treating acute Low Back Pain due to Lumbar Spondylosis.

Exercises

Exercises for low back pain are designed to relax the muscles, make them flexible and finally strengthen them.[288] The relaxation exercises release muscle tension and the stretching exercises that follow the relaxation exercises, make the muscles more flexible and thereby lengthen the key postural muscles. The strengthening exercises help the individual to overcome muscle rigidity. Exercises are useful for eliminating low back pain.[289] Those exercises fit for strengthening the muscles of the lower back should be done under the supervision of a trained practitioner. Exercise may be the last thing, the individual like to think about, when his low back is aching, but specialists say, exercise is the best thing for chronic low back pain.[290]

Physical exercises should be undertaken after due consideration of age, physical capacity, place, time and food habits, other wise it may invite disorders.[291] Weight bearing exercises such as walking, help to strengthen the

---

[288] Alexander Melleby, <u>Six Weeks to a Healthy Back</u>, Sheldon Press, London, 1990, P.7

[289] SreeKumar.P, <u>Universal Health Research,</u> Universal Press and Publications, Trivandrum, 2004, P.243.

[290] Debora Tkae, <u>The Doctor's Book on Home Remedies,</u> Parsons/ Walton Press, Hong Kong, 2001, P.40

[291] Valiathan.M.S, <u>The legacy of Susruta</u> (Quotes from Susruta cikitsa, 24-28 ,48 ½), Orient LongMan, Hyderabad 2007, P.3

bones by increasing the calcium deposits in the bones, thus increases the bone density and reduce the risk for Osteoporosis.[292] A number of different theories are used by Physical therapists to treat Low back pain. Two popular approaches are Mckenzie Extension Exercises and Williams Flexion Exercises.[293]

Sitting upright on a chair with the feet flat on the floor, roll slowly back on the sitting bones and then forward as far as the person can. Now find the mid position and familiarize with this. Lying with the knees bend, gently flatten the small of the back to the floor and hold for ten seconds. Repeat ten times. This sort of exercise reduces low back pain.[294]

Stretching techniques can be used to improve flexibility which will provide relief to low back pain.[295] Static stretching, Ballistic stretching and Proprioceptive neuromuscular facilitation are the three different types of streching methods.

Abdominal muscle control is another key to the stabilization of the low back, which in turn will reduce the back ache.[296] Physiotherapy is one of the

---

[292] STACI NIX, William's Basic Nutrition and Diet Therapy, Mosby Inc, St.Louis, Missouri, 2005, P.294

[293] Brotzman.S.B.,Clinical Orthopaedic Rehabilitation,ed2, Mosby Publishers, St.Louis, 2003, P.92

[294] John Tanner, Your Guide to Back Pain, Hodder Arnold Publishers, London, 2005, PP.155-156

[295] David.K.Miller, Measurement by the Physical Educator;Why and How., McGraw –Hill International edition, Boston, 2006, P.154.

[296] DeRosa.C., Poterfield.J., A Physical Therapy Model for the treatment of Low Back Pain., Physical Therapy, 72(4):262, 1992.

popular modes of treatment for relieving low back pain.[297] The treatment is also aimed at improving the mobility of the vertebral joints, strengthening the muscles, improving the Posture, improving blood circulation, preventing the recurrence of the pain. Today Physical Therapist embrace the new and successful medical philosophy of early active treatment of low back ache which comprise programme that include; strengthening of the muscles, flexibility exercises and aerobics.[298] Physiotherapy modalities such as Ultra sound, Transcutaneous electrical nerve stimulation (TENS), gentle spinal mobilizations can be effective, especially for localized low back pain caused due to Ankylosing spondylitis.[299]

Atlas and Nardin [300] are of the view that, for patients whose symptoms of low back ache are not improving over 2 to 4 weeks, referral for physical treatments is appropriate. When there is low back pain due to a small protrusion .of the nucleus pulposus, Traction is a treatment of choice. Through traction, the lumbar vertebrae are distracted, a sub atmospheric pressure is created; which

---

[297] Rajendra.K.V., Jindal.S.R., Rehman.A., Treat Your Spinal Problem Without Drugs, Institute of Naturopathy & Yogic Science, Bangalore, 1997, P.51.

[298] Mammen Mathew (ed.), The WEEK- Book of Healthy Living, Penguin Books Ltd, New Delhi, 2006, P.122.

[299] Bulstrode.S.J., Barefoot.J., Harrison.R., Clarke.A., The role of Passive stretching in the treatment of Ankylosing Spondylitis, Br.J.Rheumatol, 1987, 26: 40-42

[300] Atlas.S.J., Nardin.R.A., Physical Therapy for Low back ache, Muscle and Nerve Journal, 2003, Mar;27(3):265-284.

tends to pull the protrusion to it's original position.[301] Since many illnesses (including low back ache) result from the stress and strain of daily life, massage therapy is very effective as it calms and soothes tension and brings balance in human being.[302] Massage helps the flow of blood and lymph in the human body. The best intervention for the patients with Low back pain is a team approach using the skills not only of an Occupational therapist but also those of a Physician, Physiotherapist and a Psychologist.[303]

1.6 OBJECTIVES OF THE STUDY

The objectives of the study are listed below.

1. To find out the influence of yogic practices, naturopathy, physiotherapy and combined yoga & naturopathy treatments on selected dependent variable; disability index dimension - pain intensity.

2. To find out the influence of yogic practices, naturopathy, physiotherapy and combined yoga & naturopathy treatments on selected dependent variable; disability index dimension – personal care.

---

[301] Binkley.J., Finch.E., Hall.J., Diagnostic Classification of Patients with Low Back Pain, Physical Therapy, 73(3).138: 1993

[302] Sara and Thomas, Massage for Common Ailments, Gala Book Ltd, London, 1989, P.11

[303] Heidi Mellugh Pendleton, Winifred Schultz Krohn, PEDRETTI's Occupational Therapy-Practice Skills for Physical Dysfunction, (sixth edition), Mosby Publishers, New York, 2006, P.1039

3. To find out the influence of yogic practices, naturopathy, physiotherapy and combined yoga & naturopathy treatments on selected dependent variable; disability index dimension – <u>lifting.</u>

4. To find out the influence of yogic practices, naturopathy, physiotherapy and combined yoga & naturopathy treatments on selected dependent variable; disability index dimension – <u>walking.</u>

5. To find out the influence of yogic practices, naturopathy, physiotherapy and combined yoga & naturopathy treatments on selected dependent variable; disability index dimension – <u>sitting.</u>

6. To find out the influence of yogic practices, naturopathy, physiotherapy and combined yoga & naturopathy treatments on selected dependent variable; disability index dimension – <u>standing.</u>

7. To find out the influence of yogic practices, naturopathy, physiotherapy and combined yoga & naturopathy treatments on selected dependent variable; disability index dimension – <u>sleeping.</u>

8. To find out the influence of yogic practices, naturopathy, physiotherapy and combined yoga & naturopathy treatments on selected dependent variable; disability index dimension – <u>social life.</u>

9. To find out the influence of yogic practices, naturopathy, physiotherapy and combined yoga & naturopathy treatments on selected dependent variable; disability index dimension – <u>travelling.</u>

10. To find out the influence of yogic practices, naturopathy, physiotherapy and combined yoga & naturopathy treatments on selected dependent variable; disability index dimension – <u>employment/ home making.</u>

11. To find out the influence of yogic practices, naturopathy, physiotherapy and combined yoga & naturopathy treatments on <u>total disability index.</u>

12. To find out the influence of yogic practices, naturopathy, physiotherapy and combined yoga & naturopathy treatments on <u>visual analogue scale.</u>

13. To find out the influence of yogic practices, naturopathy, physiotherapy and combined yoga & naturopathy treatments on <u>spinal flexion.</u>

14. To find out the influence of yogic practices, naturopathy, physiotherapy and combined yoga & naturopathy treatments on <u>low back pain.</u>

1.7 STATEMENT OF THE PROBLEM

The present study is entitled as " the influence of Yogic practices, Naturopathy and Physiotherapy on low back pain patients ".

1.8 DELIMITATIONS OF THE STUDY

1 The study has been confined only to one hundred patients.

2 The study has been confined only to low back pain.

3 Only mild, acute and chronic low back pain were taken for the study. Complicated cases of low back pain have been excluded from the study.

4 Only selected Yogic practices, selected Naturopathic treatment and selected Physiotherapy treatment were given for the patients in the study.

5   The study has been confined for a period of three months.

1.9 LIMITATIONS OF THE STUDY

1   Factors like individual habits, life style, routine work, diet etc has affected the results of this investigation.

2   The subjects for the study, differed in weight, age, gender, geographic conditions, psychological and sociological factors.

3   It was not possible to control the daily activities of the subjects during the experiment period.

1.10 HYPOTHESES

The hypotheses framed for the present investigation are as follows:

Hypothesis 1-A

There would be significant reduction on selected dependent variable; disability index dimension - **pain intensity,** due to yogic practices, naturopathy, physiotherapy and combined yoga & naturopathy treatments.

Hypothesis 1-B

There would not be any differencial effect for the various experimental treatment groups in reducing selected dependent variable; disability index dimension - **pain intensity,** due to yogic practices, naturopathy, physiotherapy and combined yoga & naturopathy treatments.

Hypothesis 2-A

There would be significant improvement on selected dependent variable; disability index dimension – **personal care** due to yoga, naturopathy, physiotherapy and combined yoga & naturopathy treatments.

Hypothesis 2-B

There would not be any differencial effect for the various experimental treatment groups in improving selected dependent variable; disability index dimension – **personal care,** due to yogic practices, naturopathy, physiotherapy and combined yoga & naturopathy treatments.

Hypothesis 3-A

There would be significant improvement on selected dependent variable; disability index dimension – **lifting** due to yoga, naturopathy, physiotherapy and combined yoga & naturopathy treatments.

Hypothesis 3-B

There would not be any differencial effect for the various experimental treatment groups in improving selected dependent variable; disability index dimension **lifting,** due to yogic practices, naturopathy, physiotherapy and combined yoga & naturopathy treatments.

Hypothesis 4-A

There would be significant improvement on selected dependent variable; disability index dimension – **walking** due to yoga, naturopathy, physiotherapy and combined yoga & naturopathy treatments.

Hypothesis 4-B

There would not be any differencial effect for the various experimental treatment groups in improving selected dependent variable; disability index dimension–**walking,** due to yogic practices, naturopathy, physiotherapy and combined yoga & naturopathy treatments.

Hypothesis 5-A

There would be significant improvement on selected dependent variable; disability index dimension – **sitting** due to yoga, naturopathy, physiotherapy and combined yoga & naturopathy treatments.

Hypothesis 5-B

There would not be any differencial effect for the various experimental treatment groups in improving selected dependent variable; disability index dimension–**sitting,** due to yogic practices, naturopathy, physiotherapy and combined yoga & naturopathy treatments.

Hypothesis 6-A

There would be significant improvement on selected dependent variable; disability index dimension – **standing** due to yoga, naturopathy, physiotherapy and combined yoga & naturopathy treatments.

Hypothesis 6-B

There would not be any differencial effect for the various experimental treatment groups in improving selected dependent variable; disability index dimension–**standing,** due to yogic practices, naturopathy, physiotherapy and combined yoga & naturopathy treatments.

Hypothesis 7-A

There would be significant improvement on selected dependent variable; disability index dimension – **sleeping** due to yoga, naturopathy, physiotherapy and combined yoga & naturopathy treatments.

Hypothesis 7-B

There would not be any differencial effect for the various experimental treatment groups in improving selected dependent variable; disability index dimension–**sleeping,** due to yogic practices, naturopathy, physiotherapy and combined yoga & naturopathy treatments.

Hypothesis 8-A

There would be significant improvement on selected dependent variable; disability index dimension – **social life** due to yoga, naturopathy, physiotherapy and combined yoga & naturopathy treatments.

Hypothesis 8-B

There would not be any differencial effect for the various experimental treatment groups in improving selected dependent variable; disability index dimension–**social life,** due to yogic practices, naturopathy, physiotherapy and combined yoga & naturopathy treatments.

Hypothesis 9-A

There would be significant improvement on selected dependent variable; disability index dimension–**travelling** due to yoga, naturopathy, physiotherapy and combined yoga & naturopathy treatments.

Hypothesis 9-B

There would not be any differencial effect for the various experimental treatment groups in improving selected dependent variable; disability index dimension–**travelling,** due to yogic practices, naturopathy, physiotherapy and combined yoga & naturopathy treatments.

Hypothesis 10-A

There would be significant improvement on selected dependent variable; disability index dimension–**employment/home making** due to yoga, naturopathy, physiotherapy and combined yoga & naturopathy treatments.

Hypothesis 10-B

There would not be any differencial effect for the various experimental treatment groups in improving selected dependent variable; disability index dimension– **employment/home making,** due to yogic practices, naturopathy, physiotherapy and combined yoga & naturopathy treatments.

Hypothesis 11-A

There would be significant reduction on selected dependent variable; **disability index (total)** due to yoga, naturopathy, physiotherapy and combined yoga & naturopathy treatments.

Hypothesis 11-B

There would not be any differencial effect for the various experimental treatment groups in reducing selected dependent variable; **disability index (total),** due to yogic practices, naturopathy, physiotherapy and combined yoga & naturopathy treatments.

Hypothesis 12-A

There would be significant reduction on selected dependent variable; **visual analogue scale** due to yoga, naturopathy, physiotherapy and combined yoga & naturopathy treatments.

Hypothesis 12-B

There would not be any differencial effect for the various experimental treatment groups in reducing selected dependent variable; **visual analogue scale** due to yogic practices, naturopathy, physiotherapy and combined yoga & naturopathy treatments.

Hypothesis 13-A

There would be significant improvement on selected dependent variable; **spinal flexion** due to yoga, naturopathy, physiotherapy and combined yoga & naturopathy treatments.

Hypothesis 13-B

There would not be any differencial effect for the various experimental treatment groups in improving selected dependent variable; **spinal flexion** due to yogic practices, naturopathy, physiotherapy and combined yoga & naturopathy treatments.

Hypothesis 14 -A

There would be significant reduction on **low back pain** due to yoga, naturopathy, physiotherapy and combined yoga & naturopathy treatments.

Hypothesis 14 -B

There would not be any differencial effect for the various experimental treatment groups in reducing **low back pain** due to yogic practices, naturopathy, physiotherapy and combined yoga & naturopathy treatments.

1.11 DEFINITION OF KEY TERMS

Yoga

Yoga [i] is a methodised effort towards self perfection by the expression of the potentialities latent in the being and a union of the human individual with the universal and transcendent existance, we see partially expressed in man and in the cosmos.

---

[i] Kireet Joshi, <u>Philosophy and Yoga of Sri Aurobindo</u>, The Mother's Institute of Research, Mysore, 2003, P.33

Asana

Asana has been defined by Pathanjali, as that body pose, which not only confirms to steadiness, but which also is equally pleasant and comfortable.[ii]

Naturopathy

Naturopathy is a constructive method of treatment which aims at removing the basic causes of disease, through the rational use of the elements freely available in nature.[iii]

Physiotherapy

It is the treatment of disorders or injuries with physical methods or agents which is used to reduce joint stiffness and restore muscle strength.[iv]

Pain

It is defined as a subjective unpleasant sensation resulting from the stimulation of sensory nerve endings by injury, disease or other harmful factors.[v]

[ii] Yogendra, Yoga & Physical Education, The Yoga Institute Publishers, Bombay, 1956, P. 49

[iii] Bakhru.H.R., A Complete Hand book of NATURE CURE, Jaico Publishing House, Mumbai, 2006, P.3

[iv] Tony Smith, The British Medical Association, Complete Family Health Encyclopedia, Dorling Kindersley Ltd, London, 1998, P.803

[v] Mikel.A.Rothenberg, Charles.F.ChapMan, Dictionary of Medical Terms (Barron's Medical Guide), New Age International (P) Ltd Publishers, New Delhi, 2000, P.429

Low Back Pain

It is the pain affecting the lower back, often restricting the movement.[vi]

Questionnaire [vii]

It can be defined as a list of planned written questions, which are related to a particular topic or series of topics.

Oswestry Disability Questionnaire [viii]

It is a questionnaire used to assess patients with low back pain by determining it's impact on the activities of daily living.

Quadruple Visual Analogue Scale

It is a reliable and valid method for pain measurement which is based on four specific factors; the pain level at the time of the current patient visit, the typical or average pain since the last visit, the pain level at it's best, since the last visit and the pain level at it's worst, since the last visit.[ix]

[vi] Michael Peters, The British Medical Association: Illustrated Medical Dictionary, Dorling Kindersley Ltd, London, 2002, P.63

[vii] Soul.B.Herton, Choseter.L.Hunt, Sociology, McGraw Hill Inc., New York, 1976, P 99

[viii] Fairbank.JCT, Davies.JB, The Oswestry Low back Pain Disability Questionnaire, Physiotherapy, 1980, 66, 271

Modified Schober's Test

It is a method of assessing the range of lumbar spinal flexion in patients having lower back pain, by measuring the spine when the patient is errect and then bend forwards, any gain gives unequivocal evidence of spinal flexion.[x]

1.12 SCOPE AND SIGNIFICANCE OF THE STUDY

> The research findings may bring to light the effectiveness of Yogic practices, Naturopathic and Physiotherapy treatment in eliminating low back pain.

> This study may create awareness among the people about the elimination of low back pain by suitable Yogic practices, Naturopathic and Physiotherapy treatment.

> This study may create awareness among the people about the good and bad postures, which is of much significance in day to day life.

> The findings of this research may help to explore the possibilities of further research in to more acute and congenital pain in the whole back.

> The study may be of great significance to those who are involved in research in the area of Physical Education and Health Science.

[ix] Craig.E.Morris, <u>Low Back Syndromes – Integrated Clinical Management,</u> McGraw Hill (Professional) Publishing , New York, 2006, P.427

[x] Macrae.I.F, Wright.V, Measurement of Back Movement, <u>Annals of Rheumatic Diseases,</u> 1969, 28, 584-89

➢ The results of this study may be used for measuring the status and progress in fitness and also as a therapy.

Almost every person will have at least one episode of low back pain at some time in his or her life. The pain can vary from severe and long term to mild and short lived. It will resolve within a few weeks for most people. The impact of back pain on our society is enormous. It is the number one musculoskeletal condition and the number two overall health condition that cause us to seek help from the healthcare providers. The epidemic of low back pain is now made worse by growing adult and child population that is generally overweight, exercises infrequently and has poor muscle tone and posture. The lower back pain has tremendous effect on the personal lives. The psychological and emotional stress placed on the individual and their families is unimaginable. The loss of ability to participate in normal daily activities including playing with the children, to sit comfortably during a movie, sexual intimacy and a normal sleep cycle can lead to emotional mood swings and depression. It is utmost necessary that the health problem; low back pain has to be addressed in the right manner. For mild and acute lower back pain, treatment by means of yogic practices, naturopathy and physiotherapy might be beneficial. Here in this study, the investigator tries to find out, which of these treatments is most suitable for curing low back pain.

1.13 ORGANISATION OF THE REPORT

The report has been presented in five chapters. Chapter i, presents a detailed description of low back pain, yoga, naturopathy and Physiotherapy. It also describes the objectives of the study, statement of the problem, delimitations and limitations of the study, hypotheses of the study, definition of the key terms used and the scope and significance of the study.

Chapter ii, presents a detailed review of selected literature from the areas of low back pain & yoga, low back pain & naturopathy and low back pain & physiotherapy.

Chapter iii, of the thesis describes the detailed methodology. In this chapter, the selection of subjects, selection of variables, the experimental design, tools/ techniques adopted, the experimental treatment details of yoga, naturopathy and physiotherapy, the collection of data in the pre test and post test and the statistical techniques used, are narrated.

The detailed analysis of the data collected and it's interpretation, discussion of the hypotheses and tenability and discussion on the findings are given in chapter iv.

A short overlook of the study, major findings, suggestions and suggestions for further research are given in chapter v.

Chapter ii

REVIEW
OF LITERATURE

Chapter ii

REVIEW OF RELATED LITERATURE

2.1 INTRODUCTION

Familiarity with the literature related to any problem helps the investigator to discover what is already known and what others have attempted to find out, what methods of approach have been promising or disappointing and what problems remain to be solved. The review would enable the investigator to have a deep insight, clear perspective and a better understanding of a chosen problem and the various factors connected with the study.

According to Aggarwal, "The literature in any field forms the foundation upon which all future work will be built ".[1]

Best [2] says; Research is the most systematic activity directed towards the discovery and the development of an organized body of knowledge.

A study of relevant literature is an essential step to get a good comprehension of what has been done with regard to the problem under study. Such a review will bring in a new sight and will help in the development of

---

[1] Aggarwal.J.C, <u>Educational Research</u>, Arya Book Depot, New Delhi, 1975, P.109

[2] John.W. Best; <u>Research in Education</u>, Prentice Hall Inc., New Jersey, 1977, P.16

research procedures. The investigator has attempted in this chapter to locate relevant literature related to this study.

2.2 STUDIES RELATED TO YOGA AND LOW BACK PAIN

Sherman[3] and colleagues compared how yoga, therapeutic exercise, and a self-help book affected chronic low back pain. The randomized controlled trial included adults who were diagnosed with low back pain and were recruited via health plan magazine advertisements and direct mailings. Patients were excluded if they reported minimal pain (0 to 2 points on a severity scale, with 10 being the highest level of pain) or if a specific underlying condition was the confirmed or likely cause of pain. Patients were also excluded if they were receiving physical therapy for back pain, had serious medical or psychiatric conditions, or had work schedules that were incompatible with the class schedule. The 101 participants were predominantly women (66 percent), had some college education (97 percent), and were employed (87 percent). Sixty-seven percent of participants reported pain lasting more than one year.

Participants were randomly assigned to an intention-to-treat intervention (i.e., 12 weekly, 75-minutes yoga classes, 12 weekly 75-minute exercise classes, or an evidence-based self-help book containing strategies for managing back

---

[3] Karen.J.Sherman, Yoga improves chronic low back pain, Annnals of Internal Medicine, 20th Dec.2005, Vol.143, (12), 849-856.

pain). One instructor led each of the exercise and yoga classes. Yoga classes consisted of breathing exercises, a sequence of postures designed to relieve low back symptoms and guided relaxation. Exercise classes consisted of gradually increasing aerobic repetitions and strengthening exercises followed by stretching. Participants who received self-help books had no instructions and did not attend classes. Information about functional status, which was based on a 24-point Roland Disability Scale, and on symptom severity, which was based on an 11-point "bothersomeness" scale, was gathered by telephone interviews at 6, 12, and 26 weeks. Participants in the yoga and exercise groups had similar class attendance with participants attending 9 of the 12 classes, on average. Eighty-seven percent of participants in the self-help group reported reading at least one third of the book. Ninety-five participants completed the 26-week interview.

Although functionality and symptom severity improved in all groups, the yoga group had the best results. At 26 weeks (14 weeks after the completion of classes), the yoga group's mean disability score was 3.6 points lower than that of the self-help group and 1.5 points lower than that of the exercise group (2.5 points was considered clinically significant). Similarly, the yoga group's mean symptom score was 2.2 points lower than that of the self-help group and 1.4 points lower than that of the exercise group (1.5 points was considered clinically significant). In addition, reported pain medication use in the week preceding the week 26 interview was significantly lower in the yoga group (21 percent) than in the exercise group (50 percent) or self-help group (59 percent). The investigators concluded that yoga was more effective than a self-help book for treating chronic low back pain, producing clinical benefits at least equivalent to, and possibly better than, traditional therapeutic exercise.

Moorthy and Videmen[4] conducted a study on the influence of Yogic practices for the treatment of low back pain. Twenty two men in the age group of 30-45 years were selected as subjects. They were suffering from non specific lumbar back pain. All the subjects were administered with spinal disorder quistionnaire, mood variables and selected spinal mobility variable before and after the experiment. The Yogic training programme (which consists of Ardh-Salabasana, Bhujangasana, Naukasana, Dhanurasana, Ekapada Pavanamukthasana and Janusirasana) was provided in the evening for one hour daily and for a period of 12 weeks. After the experiment period, they found out that low back pain has been reduced considerably in the subjects.

In order to assess the effectiveness of yoga therapy on the cure of low back ache, Kieok[5] conducted a study in Therapeutic Hospital at Nashik, India, in association with Yoga Vidya Gurukul of Nashik. His study consisted of 60

---

[4] Moorthy.A.M., Videmen, Influence of different types of Exercise for the treatment of Low back Pain,(Abstracts), International Conference, CSS Haryana Agricultural University, 1995, P.44-49

[5] Chong Chiew Kieok, Yoga cures low back ache, Current Reviews in Musculoskeletal Medicine, Vol.1, No.1, Mar.2008, 39-47

low back pain patients, out of which 30 patients were given yoga treatment and the other 30 patients were treated with natural homeopathy consisted of some homeopathic medicines, massage and steam bath. Massage was given twice a day, once each in the morning and evening for 30-day sessions. The patients were over 40 years of age, with majority of them aged around 50-60 years old. Approximately three-quarters (70%-75%) of the back ache patients were females, and most of these patients were working in the office, travelling job or travellers on 2-wheelers. Approximately 60% of the patients with back pain were due to obesity. The Yoga treatment given by Kieok was a monthly course of an hour daily yoga session consisted of asanas like Noukasana, Bhujangasana, Merudandasana, Salabhasana, Janusirasana, Leghu Pavanamukthasana and Vakrasana along with pranayama. The patients practiced pranayama 21 times (approximately 5 minutes) daily. When assessed by Oswestry disability scores after the experiment, the Yoga group had much more improvement than the Homeo group (p less than 0.004). Visual analogue pain scores also showed significant reduction in pain for the Yoga group. The study concluded that yogasanas could be effective for low back ache that are caused by factors such as obesity, improper sitting posture, strains of muscles, and lumber scoliosis. However, for back ache caused by old sport injuries, the effectiveness of yogasanas need further research, both in terms of the types of asanas to be practiced as well as the type of injuries to be considered. The findings from the case study indicated that a backache-free life could be expected for those who treat yoga as a routine in their daily life.

Angamuthu[6] has studied the influence of selected yogic practices and physical exercises on low back pain patients. Ninety male low back pain patients, aged between 25–50 years, were randomly selected from school-college teachers, transport workers, Head load workers and Merchants in Tamil Nadu. They have been divided in to three groups of 30 each; Yoga group, Physical exercise group and control group. Ransford et al low back pain questionnaire has been used to assess the pain before the experiment and after the experiment. Yoga group had been provided with selected yogic exercises which included Salabhasana, Dhanurasana, Janusirasana, Uthanapadasana, Pavanamukthasana, Noukasana and Bhujangasana for one hour daily and for a period of 12 weeks. The physical exercise group has been provided with exercises which included Prone back lift, Hand and Shoulder curl, Alternate leg extension, Lower the legs exercise, Sitting tucks, Modified sit ups, Half knee bend and Toe touching. The duration of these exercises was also one hour daily and for a period of 12 weeks. The control group was kept idle, with out any yogic practices/ exercises. It has been found that low back pain has been reduced much, in yoga group than physical exercise and control groups.

Gharote[7] conducted a study on the "effects of yogic training on physical fitness" and discovered that physical fitness could be achieved by way of yogic

---

[6] Kandasamy Angamuthu, Influence of Yogic practices and Physical exercises on low back pain patients, <u>Ph.D Thesis, Alagappa University,</u> Tamil Nadu, 1999.

practices. For the study, he has selected 27 males and 12 females who were undergoing a course in yoga practices. Twenty different asanas were given to the subjects for a period of three weeks. For the assessment of physical fitness, comprehensive tests were administered before the experiment and after the experiment and data were drawn. Statistical analysis of the data collected showed that yogic practices considerably improved physical fitness.

Williams and Petronis [8] have conducted a research by a randomized control trial in subjects with non-specific chronic low back pain, comparing Iyengar yoga therapy to an educational control group. Both programs were 16 weeks long. Subjects were primarily self-referred and screened by primary care physicians for study of inclusion/exclusion criteria. The primary outcome for the study was functional disability. Secondary outcomes including present pain intensity, pain medication usage, pain-related attitudes and behaviors, and spinal range of motion were measured before and after the interventions. Subjects had low back pain for 11.2±1.54 years and 48% used pain medication. Overall, subjects presented with less pain and lower functional disability than subjects in other published intervention studies for chronic low back pain. Of the 60

---

[7] Gharote.M.L., Effect of Yogic training on Physical Fitness, <u>Yogamimamsa:</u>15 (1973), P. 43.

[8] Kimberly Anne Williams, John Petronis, Iyengar Yoga & Chronic Low back Pain, <u>Pain,</u> Vol.115, Issues 1-2, May 2005, 107-117

subjects enrolled, 42 (70%) completed the study. Multivariate analyses of outcomes in the categories of medical, functional, psychological and behavioral factors indicated that significant differences between groups existed in functional and medical outcomes but not for the psychological or behavioral outcomes. Univariate analyses of medical and functional outcomes revealed significant reductions in pain intensity (64%), functional disability (77%) and pain medication usage (88%) in the yoga group at the post and 3-month follow-up assessments. These preliminary data indicated that the majority of self-referred persons with mild chronic low back pain would comply to and report improvement on medical and functional pain-related outcomes from Iyengar yoga therapy.

Galantino, Bzdewka and Russo [9] have conducted a randomized study, the purpose of which was to evaluate a possible design for a 6-week modified Hatha yoga protocol (yoga with pranayama) and to study the effects on participants with chronic low back pain. Twenty two participants (M = 5; F = 17), between the ages of 30 and 65, with chronic low back pain (CLBP) were randomized to either an immediate yoga based intervention, or to a control group with no treatment during the observation period, but received later yoga training. The methods included a specific CLBP yoga protocol designed and modified for this

---

[9] Galantino.M.L, Bzdewka.T.M, Eissler-Russo.J.L, <u>Alternative Therapies in Health and Medicine.</u> 2004 Mar-Apr;10(2):56-59

population by a certified yoga instructor, which was administered for one hour, twice a week for 6 weeks. Primary functional outcome measures included the forward reach (FR) and sit and reach (SR) tests. All participants completed Oswestry Disability Index (ODI) and Beck Depression Inventory (BDI) questionnaires. Guiding questions were used for qualitative data analysis to ascertain how yoga participants perceived the instructor, group dynamics, and the impact of yoga on their life. To account for drop outs, the data were divided into 'better or not' categories, and analyzed using chi-square to examine differences between the groups. Qualitative data were analyzed through frequency of positive responses. Potentially important trends in the functional measurement scores showed improved balance and flexibility and decreased disability and depression for the yoga group. The researchers concluded that a modified yoga-based intervention benefit individuals with Chronic Low Back Pain.

Graves et al,[10] have studied Hatha yoga (yoga with pranayama) and found out that it is valuable for preventing and managing stress-related chronic health problems, including low back pain. In a survey of 3000 people receiving yoga for health ailments (1142 [38%] with back pain), 98% claimed that yoga benefited them. The investigators also reported that in a case series of 16 patients using various asanas for rehabilitation, 11 (69%) reported significant

---

[10] Nathan Graves et al, Yoga & Stress related health problems, <u>The Journal of Family Practice,</u> August 2004, Vol. 53, No. 8

improvement, with near normal mobility and absence of pain. Those who reported recurring back pain also reported irregular practice of yoga. In another case series, 21 women aged $\geq$60 years (mean age, 75) with hyperkyphosis, participated in twice-weekly 1-hour sessions of hatha yoga for 12 weeks. Measured height increased by a mean of 0.52 cm, forward curvature diminished, patients were able to get out of chairs faster, and they had longer functional reach. Eleven patients (48%) reported increased postural awareness/ improvement and improved well-being; 58% perceived improvement in their physical functioning.

Miller [11] has studied the impact of yogic practices on patients who were suffering from low back pain (sciatica) for about three years. The patients felt constant twinges in their lower back due to scoliosis, or curvature of the spine. They have been administered yogic practices suitable for Scoliosis (yoga to work with the reverse-S curve of their spine). For the next month they took time off to devote themselves to healing. Within four weeks they were sleeping without pain, and the daily pain wasn't as dominant. About a month after that, the daily pain ended. Not only that, the patients believed that the curve in their lower back was lessening. They got complete recovery from the sciatica by practicing selected Yogasanas.

---

[11] Elise Miller, Impact of yogic practices on Scoliosis, <u>Yoga Journal</u>, May/Jun 2001, P.40.

Vad [12] launched "Back Builders," a new program combining yoga, breath-work, and Pilates to help patients to heal from disk injuries. He says; "Lower back pain is really a mind-body problem, closely related to stress." He formulated a program that combines the mind and body components. Twenty-five program participants practiced a series of poses and exercises, mostly supine, three times a week at home while they were still largely immobilized by their injuries. Later they participated in a more challenging 'Back Builders' class three times a week at Practice Yoga studio in Manhattan. The basic idea behind "Back Builders" is to build core strength and flexibility and lengthen the spine to create space between the vertebrae, thus minimizing pressure on the disks and allowing them to heal. The program emphasizes asanas that build support for the spine by strengthening the abdominal and back muscles. The classic hip-opening poses encourage spinal length, as do postures that stretch the hamstrings and calves. Participants also did gentle back extension exercises.

Vad also followed a second group of 25 disk-injury patients who did not participated in the yoga program. Both groups took the pain medications. After six months Vad found remarkable results; 80 percent of those in the Back Builders program experienced markedly decreased pain, compared with 44 percent of those on medications only. The yoga also seemed to help in

---

[12] Vijay Vad, Hilary Hinzmann, <u>BACK Rx – A 15 minute – a- Day Yoga & Pilates-Based Programme to end Low Back Pain</u>, Gotham Books, New York, 2004, PP.126 - 129

preventing recurrences. Only 12 percent of the yoga practitioners experienced another acute episode of their injury, compared with 56 percent of those on medications alone. Also, the pain medication use of those doing yoga declined by 40 percent.

Vidhyasagar [13] et al have conducted research on the effects of Hatha yoga on non specific chronic low back pain. They have selectd 35 patients and administered classical back bending postures of yoga for a duration of 45 minutes daily with 10 minutes rest in between the poses and for a period of three weeks. The poses modified in the case of 5 subjects because of severe pain to include Pavanamukthasana and Ardha Uttanasana in phase 1. The researchers concluded that 76% of the subjects got pain relief.

Beckman Bee[14] has conducted research on the effect of various yogasanas on bone mineral density and body composition in adult women and discovered that bone mineral density increased significantly in the spine in the experimental group who have been administered with Triangle pose, Half Moon, Extended Side Angle, and Warrior I and II poses. There was no significant change in the control group and no significant change in body composition in either the Yoga

---

[13] Vidhyasagar et al, Yoga and Chronic Low back pain, Clinical Proceedings, NIMS, Hyderabad, 1989, 4:160

[14] Phil Catalfo, Yoga & Osteoporosis, Yoga Journal, May/Jun 2001

group or the control group. The investigator concluded that osteoporosis and the resultant low back pain could be treated through regular weight bearing exercise. Yoga is an excellent weight bearing exercise as it stimulates bone building for both the upper and lower body while being low-impact.

Mukunda Stiles[15] discovered that Bhujangasana, Ardhasalabhasana, Janusirasana, Virabhadrasana and Parsvottanasana have the ability to cure pain due to tension in the lower back (scoliosis). The study has been conducted for a period of six months in patients with lumbar discomfort and weak musculature. All the asanas were given in the form of repitations and found that the practice of the above said asanas completely cured low back pain.

Karmananda Saraswathy[16] has found out that Selected Asanas; Pavanamukthasana,Vajrasana, Salabhasana, Dhanurasana and Noukasana, have curative effect on low back pain. He has conducted research on patients suffering from low back ache with the above said asanas and each has been practiced for 12 minutes in the morning without fail, followed by 10 minutes in Savasana for a duration of 12 weeks. This programme was specially designed to increase the functional effeciency of the various muscle groups responsible for low back pain.

---

[15] Mukunda Stiles, <u>Structural Yoga Therapy</u>, GoodWill Publishing House, New Delhi, 2002, PP. 267-268.

[16] Karmananda Saraswathy Swamy, <u>Yogic Management of Common Diseases</u>, Bihar School of Yoga, Munger, Bihar, 1983, P.148

De Vries [17] evaluated the strategic stretching procedures of Hatha Yoga for improvement of flexibility. He has selected Fifty seven college students, who were divided into two groups; one of the group has been trained by static stretching of Hatha yoga and the other group by conventional ballistic methods of stretching for thirty minutes a day and for a period of seven weeks. Both the groups made statistically significant gains, when measured by flexibility tests. However it has been revealed that the static stretching method of Hata yoga seems preferable.

Moorthy[18] in his study, has discovered that Yogasanas improved flexibility. He did an experimental study of 90 boys and equal no.of girls by giving training in specific asanas for six weeks. After the training period, the change in flexibility had been by judged by Cureton's flexibility test. Among Asanas, Bhujangasana has been found very effective, which controls and relaxes the muscles and improves it's elasticity.

Several studies have been conducted to assess the effect of Yogic practices on low back pain patients. The studies conducted by Flint[19],

---

[17] Herbert A De Vries, Evaluation of static stretching procedures for the improvement of flexibility, Research Quarterly, 33:2.222 – 229 (1962)

[18] Moorthy.A.M., Effect of selected Yogasanas and Physical Exercises on Flexibility, Yoga Review,Vol.11,316 (1982)

[19] Marilin Flint.M, Effect of increasing back and abdominal muscle strength on low back pain patients, Santa Barbara College Journal, University of California, 2001, P.41

Mahadevan[20],Graves and Krepcho[21], Bhaskara Menon[22], Kenneth[23], Clara[24], Kuvalayananda and Vinekar[25], Donald Norfolk [26], Jane Hart [27], Jones Mecarthy [28], Nithin Gorpal and Ganesh Shankar[29], Mishra[30], Frawley[31], Steinberg and Petronis[32], Lively[33], Sorovsky and Stilp[34], Sturgess[35], Niranjananda[36] and

---

[20] Mahadevan, Effects of selected physical Exercises and Yogasanas on the spinal mobility of aged Sports Men, SNIPES journal, July 1993, P.52

[21] Graves, Krepcho, Mayo, Hill ; Effectiveness of yoga for low back pain, Journal of Family Practice, Vol 53(8):661-62. August 2004,

[22] Bhaskara Menon.K.P.(Yoga Retna), Yogasanas and Miracles, Life Yoga Centre, Kochi, 2002, PP.31-39

[23] Kenneth.W.Lin.,Therapeutic Exercise & Yoga on Low back pain, American Family Physician, June 1, 2006

[24] Joseph Clara.A.A., Effect of Selected yogic practices on low back pain among working women, unpublished M.Phil dissertation, Annamalai University, Tamil Nadu, 1997.

[25] Kuvalayananda Swamy, Vinekar.S.L, Yogic Therapy- it's basic Principles and Methods, Central Health Education Bureau, Directorate General of Heath Services, Govt.of India, New Delhi, 1963, P.96

[26] Donald Norfolk, Conquering Back Pain, Blandford Press, London, 1997, PP.69-70.

[27] Jane Hart, An Overview of Clinical Applications of Therapeutic Yoga, Alternative & Complimentary Therapies, Feb:2008, 14(1):29-32

[28] Jones Mecarthy, Yoga –The Way of Life, Rider & Company, London, 1969, P.28.

[29] Nitin Korpal, Ganesh Shankar, Hatha Yoga for Human Health, Satyam Publishing House, New Delhi, 2005, P.170

[30] Mishra.J.P.N., YOGA For Common Ailments, B.Jain Publishers (Pvt) Ltd, New Delhi, 1999, P.202

[31] David Frawley, Yoga and Ayurveda; Self Healing and Self Realization, Motilal Banarsidass Publishers, New Delhi, 2000, P.163

[32] Lois Steinberg, John Petronis. Therapeutic application of Iyengar Yoga for healing chronic low back pain. International Journal of Yoga Therapy, 2003, No.13, PP. 55-67.

Chidhambaran[37] had proved that Yogic practices have curative effect on low back pain patients.

2.3 STUDIES RELATED TO NATUROPATHY AND LOW BACK PAIN

Cooley, Szczurko and Bernhardt [38] have conducted a study to evaluate the effectiveness of naturopathic treatments on chronic low back pain. Naturopathic treatment as a whole is evaluated using a randomized controlled trial approach with functional outcomes within an industrialized setting. The Objectives were to evaluate the effectiveness of a combination of acupuncture treatment, lifestyle and dietary counselling, and the application of mind-body therapy in order to establish the effect of naturopathic medical treatment on disability, pain management and quality of life in chronic low back pain patients. 75 employees

---

[33] Lively.M.W., Sports Medicine Approach to Low Back Pain, Southern Medical Journal, 2002, 95.642-646

[34] Susan Sorovsky, Sonja Stilp, Yoga and it's therapeutic effect, Current Reviews in Musculoskeletal Medicine, Vol.1, No.1, Mar.2008, 39-47

[35] Stephen Sturgess, The Yoga Book – A Practical Guide to Self Realization, Motilal Banarsidass Publishers, New Delhi, 2004, P.152

[36] Niranjananda Saraswathy Swami, Yoga Darshan, Sri Panchadashnum Paramahamsa Alakh Bara, Deoghar, Bihar, 1993, P.56

[37] Chidhambaran.T.G,(Yogacharya), Yogic Practices and Treatment, Manolokam Group Publishing Co, Calicut, Kerala, 1989, P.93

[38] http://www.drhalbrown.com/Naturopathic study of LBP.php; retrieved on 16th August 2007.

of the Canadian Postal department who were suffering from mild to severe back pain of atleast 6 weeks duration volunteered to participate in this study. Oswestry, Roland and Morris (low back disability indexes), and SF-36 (quality of life) questionnaires and a pain scale were completed to assess baseline back health, pain levels and quality of life. Baseline pain medication and adjunctive therapy use, as well as lumbar length on maximum forward flexion were established. Participants were randomly selected for treatment groups, resulting in 39 active group and 36 control group participants.

The control group received bi-monthly instruction on lumbar stretching and strengthening exercises, and was encouraged to perform relaxation exercises based on a Back Pain information booklet shown previously to be equivalent to physiotherapy. Focus of the book was on education, causes of low back pain, coping strategies and encouragement to stay active.

The active group received a twice weekly standard acupuncture protocol, lifestyle advice and anti-inflammatory dietary suggestions emphasizing nutrients that promote muscle relaxation and repair (essential fatty acids, calcium/magnesium, eliminating pro-inflammatory substances such as methylxanthenes, and vegetables from the night-shade family). Relaxation techniques were performed, as were stretching exercises and activities from the back pain book as implemented in the control group. Efforts were made to give a standardized, generalized treatment with room for individualized variation.

Oswestry, Roland and Morris, SF-36, and Pain Scale questionnaires were repeated at 4, 8, and 12 weeks. At those times forward lumbar flexion and weight were recorded. Medication and therapy use was recorded at each visit. 13 participants were self-selected from the control group to undergo 4 weeks of crossover naturopathic treatment with evaluation following.

The researchers concluded that Naturopathic treatment was shown to have significant (95% CI) benefit in decreasing disability and pain due to chronic low back pain. Pain medication use was significantly reduced, and quality of life measures dramatically improved. Crossover data as well as chronological analysis of the outcomes showed the most significant changes occured within the first 4 weeks of Naturopathic treatment.

A Randomised controlled trial [39] was conducted with 240 clients aged between 20 and 65 presenting at ten general practitioners in Brent, in the summer of 2000 with low back pain of over three months duration. The experiment was with random allocation and the interventions were, Questionnaire inquiry of disability, pain and sense of well being administered at recruitment, 3, 6, 12 months, and at 5 years. Half of them, randomised to an intervention arm that comprises treatment at the British College of Naturopathy and Osteopathy (BCNO) by third/ fourth year students under the supervision of experienced trainer practitioners. This intervention was naturopathic osteopathy and included patient diaries. Upto seven treatments had been given, expecting an average of five weekly treatments. The primary outcome measures were; assessment of the Disability using the Roland Morris Score, Self competence

---

[39] http//www.naturopathicosteopathy.com, retrieved on 05th Jan.2008

using the Perceived Pain management competence scale, Beliefs using the Back Beliefs Questionnaire, Pain using the Von Korff questionnaire, Well-being using the SF-12. All of these were self-administered questionnaires. It has been concluded that naturopathic Osteopathy has positive effect on curing Low Back Pain.

Haas et al[40] have conducted a study to evaluate the effectiveness of Naturopathic Treatment in chronic low back pain patients. The design of the study was a randomized controlled trial. The subjects were community-dwelling seniors (n = 40) aged 60 and older with chronic Low Back Pain of mechanical origin. 20 Patients were randomly allocated to the Naturopathic treatment which include naturopathic diet of uncooked/partly cooked green vegetables and fresh fruits, Herbal drink, Spinal bath, Hip bath, Sun bath and light aerobic exercises and the other 20 patients to the control group for whom no treatment was given. The treatment program was for 12 weeks. Outcomes were evaluated using 100-point modified Von Korff pain and disability scale and SF-36 general health. It has been concluded by the researchers that there was considerable reduction in pain for the experiment group than the control group. The naturopathic treatment group experienced a statistically significant (P=.004) reduction in pain over the study period.

---

[40] M.Haas et al, Low back pain and Naturopathic treatment, <u>Journal of Manipulative and Physiological Therapeutics</u>, Volume 24, Issue 4, pp.117-119

Thomas Malieckal [41] has studied the influence of naturopathic treatment on low back pain patients and discovered that naturopathic diet, Sun bath, Spinal bath, Hip bath, fasting, mud therapy, prayer therapy, meditation, counseling and massage are very much useful for back pain patients. He has treated 15 patients as part of a study in his "Nature Cure Hospital, Moozhikkulam" by providing hip bath, spinal bath, massage, mud therapy, diet that consisted of whole grain foods, fresh fruits and vegetables. The patients were given pineapple which contains Bromelian, an enzyme which is very much required for strengthening of the bones. He administered calcium rich naturopathic food items to the patients. After the experiment period of 2 months, the patients showed considerable recovery from low back pain.

Herman et al [42] have conducted a study in which, Workers aged 25 to 65 years with clinical diagnosis of low-back pain of at least 6 weeks' duration were recruited from a warehouse site of a large corporation. Seventy-five participants were randomly assigned to receive 3 months of 30-minute, semi-weekly, onsite naturopathic-care visits (exercise and dietary advice, relaxation training, and a back-care educational booklet) or 3 months of 30-minute, bi-weekly, onsite control-group visits (standardized physiotherapy advice and the back-care

---

[41] Thomas Malieckal, <u>What is Nature Cure</u>, Nature Cure Hospital, Moozhikkulam, Kerala, 1987, pp.46-48

[42] Herman.P.M.et al, Efficacy of Naturopathic treatment on low back patients, <u>Alternative Therapies in Health and Medicine</u>, March/April 2008, 14(2). 32 - 39

educational booklet). All participants were told to continue their pain medications as needed. Participants' use of other adjunctive care (chiropractic care, massage, physiotherapy) was monitored. At the end of the experiment, it has been found that low back pain has been reduced considerably in naturopathic-care participants. Conversely, control-group participants had a slightly increased low back ache and tended to increase adjunctive care. The naturopathic-care group experienced a statistically significant (P=.006) increase in quality-of-life years over the study period; but the control group did not.

Jayakumar [43] has discovered that, the main causes of low back pain are muscular tension, joint strain, poor posture and incorrect nutrition resulting from dietetic errors and lack of exercises. Other causes include stress and strain resulting from sitting for a long time, improper lifting of weights, high heels and emotional problems, which cause painful cramping. Sleeping on too soft a mattress which results in an improper back and neck posture and cause tension and pain in the low back. He has conducted a study in which 12 low back pain patients were subjected to naturopathic treatment and exercise modules. The diet consisted of a salad of raw vegetables such as tomato, carrot, cabbage,

---

[43] Jayakumar.K.R., <u>Nature Cure and Yoga practices</u>, Jeevan Books, Kottayam, Kerala, 1989, P.55

cucumber, radish and two steamed or lightly cooked vegetables such as cauliflower, spinach and plenty of fruits (except bananas). Hot fomentations, alternate sponging or application of radient heat to the lower back also have been provided to the subjects. The aerobic exercise given to the subjects has improved the supply of nutrients to spinal discs, thereby delaying the process of deterioration that comes with age and eventually affects the spinal motion. After the experiment period of 12 weeks , the patients of the naturopathy group showed much reduction in their pain intensity than the control group, to whom few back exercises only provided..

Gagnier [44] and collegues looked at randomized controlled trials of the three herbals that involved nearly 1,600 adults with acute. sub-acute or chronic low back pain. The studies have been conducted by using pitted devil's claw (Harpago procumbens), white willow bark (Salix alba) and cayenne (Capsicum frutescens) against sham pills and against the painkiller. "The results of these 10 trials suggested that specific herbal medicines are effective for short-term (four to six weeks) improvement in pain and functional status for individuals with acute episodes of chronic non-specific low-back pain," the researchers concluded. "These herbal medicines could be considered as treatment options for acute episodes of chronic low back pain," they said.

---

[44] http://www.newstarget.com/019672.html; retrieved, 15th Nov.2007

Ingels [45] has conducted research and the findings of his study suggest that vitamin D deficiency is an underlying cause for persistent low back pain.The study was conducted in Saudi Arabia, where, despite the excessive sunlight, people were found deficient of Viamin D. Here most people stay indoors and cover their bodies for cultural reasons, which might be a pre-disposing factor for developing vitamin D deficiency. Deficiency of vitamin D leads to softening of the bones (osteomalacia) in adults. The author concluded that chronic low back pain may be due to osteomalacia. Vitamin D is necessary for maintaining a normal blood concentration of calcium; as it enhances the absorption of calcium from the intestine. Vitamin D is manufactured in the body from a precursor molecule that is produced when the skin is exposed to direct sunlight. Only a small amount of sun exposure is required to prevent vitamin D deficiency.

Study conducted by Norfolk [46] has revealed that naturopathic diet which contains adequate quantum of Vitamin C, Vitamin D and Calcium, reduced low back pain by assisting in the formation of sturdy bones and healthy joint tissues. His study involved 20 low back pain patients of 40 to 60 years old, who had deficiency in the intake of Vitamin C, Vitamin D and Calcium. On naturopathy

---

[45] Darin Ingels, Vitamin D; Effective Treatment for Chronic Low Back Pain, <u>Spine,</u> 2003; 28:177–179.

[46] Donald Norfolk, <u>Conquering Back Pain,</u> Blandford Press, London, 1997, PP.62-63

diet, the patients with low back pain enjoy a beneficial increase in vitamin C, vitamin D and Calcium. The subjects were given fresh citrous fruits which contains lot of vitamin C everyday, together with plenty of salads and lightly cooked vegetables like Cabbage, Beet Root and Carrot. Almond and Walnut which contain lot of calcium had also been given to the subject under study. After the experiment period of 12 weeks, Norfolk discovered that the subjects have experienced a reduction in pain in their low back.

Several studies have been conducted to assess the effect of naturopathic treatment on low back pain patients. The studies conducted by Bakhru[47], Devassy[48], Neelakandan Namboothiri[49], Jean Carper[50], Rajeev Sharma[51], Gopalakrishna Pillai & Velayudhan Nair[52], Hitendra[53], Pistina Padayattil[54],

---

[47] Bakhru.H.K, A complete hand book of Nature Cure, Jaico publishing House, Mumbai 1991, PP. 213-215.

[48] Davassy.P.P, Swayam Chikitsa (Self Treatment), Free Nature Cure service Centre, Kalady, Kerala, 2000, P.35

[49] Neelakandan Namboothiri.N.P., Home Medical Guide, Dharmacharya Publishers, Kozhikode, Kerala, 2007, P.206

[50] Jean Carper, FOOD – Your Miracle Medicine, Simon & Schuster UK Ltd, London, 1994, P.457

[51] Rajeev Sharma, A complete guide of Naturopathy, Indiana Publishing House, New Delhi 2006, PP.540-542

Swaminathan[55], Ranjith Roy[56] and Ann Louise[57] have substantiated the effectiveness of Naturopathic treatment on low back pain patients.

2.4 STUDIES RELATED TO PHYSIOTHERAPY AND LOW BACK PAIN

Shealy and Borgmeyer [58] have studied the effect of lumbar Traction on twenty low back pain patients, who were suffering from lumbar herniated disc and facet joint arthrosis. The aim of the study was to do before and after MRI to

---

[52] Gopalakrishna Pillai.K., Velayudhan Nair,(Vaidya Retnam), Health Encyclopaedia, Aradhana Publications, Shornur, Kerala, 2002, P.126

[53] Hitendra Ahooja, Herbal and Yogic remedies for Common Ailments, Wisdom Tree Publishers, New Delhi, 2002, P.9

[54] Pristeena Padayattil (Sr.), Nature Cure and Food Habits, Nature Cure Hospital, Moozhikkulam, Kerala, 1987, P.14

[55] Swaminathan.M., Hand Book of Food & Nutrition, The Bangalore Printing and Publishing Co.Ltd, Bangalore, 2006, P.89

[56] Ranjit Roy Chowdhary, UtonMuchtar Rafei, Report of World Health Organization Regional Office for South East Asia, New Delhi, 2002, P.286

[57] Ann Louise GITTELMAN, The Fat Flush Plan, Tata McGraw-Hill Publishing Company, New Delhi, 2004, P.181

[58] Shealy.C.N., Borgmeyer.V., Traction gives Relief to Low Back Pain, AMJ. Pain Management 1997,7:63-65

correlate clinical improvement with any MM evidence of disc repair in annulus, nucleus, facet joint or foramen as a result of traction treatment. A course of 20 traction treatments were given in 4 to 5 weeks to 18 patients, and a double course of 40 in 10 weeks to 2 more. Pull of distraction was adjusted to one half-body weight plus IO lbs. Each session consisted of 20 repetitions in 30 minutes of full distraction for 60 seconds and 30 seconds of relaxation to 50 lbs. Distraction angle on pelvic harness was varied from 10% for L5-S I to 20 to 25% for L4-5 herniations and above. Subjects comprised 12 males and 8 females from age 26 to 74. Radiculopathy in 14 patients was from herniated discs of varying sizes. (L5-S I level in 6, L4-5 in 6, and 1 each at L3-4 and L2-3). Radiculopathy without disc herniation was present in 6 patients from foraminal stenosis, facet arthropathy and lateral spinal stenosis. EMGs confirmed radiculopathy in all. MRI's before and after were obtained on high and mid field units. Clinical status was assessed before, during, and after treatment with standard analog pain rating scale of 0- I0 and a neuro examination. Range of motion for spinal mobility (initially impaired in all), myotomal weakness reflex and dermatomal sensory loss were tested.

In MRI outcomes, Disc Herniation; 10 of 14 improved significantly, some globally, some at least local at the site of the nerve root compression. Measured improvement in local or general disc herniation size varied in range of 0% in 2 patients, 20% in 4 patients, 30 to 50% in 4 patients and a remarkable 90 % in 2 patients who had the number of treatments at 40 sessions in 8 weeks. In clinical outcomes, irrespective of MRI status, all but 3 patients had very significant pain relief, complete relief of weakness when present, and of immobility and of all numbness. With disc herniation, 10 patients of 14 had 10 to 90% improvement in pain and disability. Two had 40 to 50%, one had only 20% with foraminal syndrome without herniation, 4 had 70 to 100 % improvement, one had 40 to 50 %, one with severe spinal stenosis had only 25%. Degree of clinical improvement roughly followed MRI changes but not totally with full correlation. Relief of pain and disability by reduction of disc size is easy to argue in a small majority of this series. A few patients had dramatic anatomic improvement. Also, many patients improved very early in treatment, probably before MRI change could be seen. The researchers concluded that Traction treatment afforded good or excellent relief of pain and disability whether from herniated disc or foraminal or lateral spinal stenosis. MRI showed imperfect correlation with degree of clinical improvement but 10 to 90% reduction in disc herniation size could be seen at least at the critical point of nerve root impingement in 10 of 14 patients. Two patients with extended courses of treatment showed 90% disc reduction.

Hurley et al [59] have conducted research to determine the efficacy of interferential therapy (IFT) - electrode placement technique compared with a

---

[59] Hurley.D.A. et al , Interferential therapy- Electrode placement technique in acute low back pain, Archives of Physical Medicine and Rehabilitation, 2001 Apr ; 82(4):485-93

control treatment in subjects with acute low back pain. The design of the study was single-blind, randomized, controlled trial with a 3-months follow-up. A random sample of 60 eligible patients from the outpatient physiotherapy departments in hospital and university settings with low back pain (28 men, 32 women) were recruited by general practitioners and self-referral for physiotherapy treatment and randomly assigned to 1 of 3 groups. The interventions were; (1) "IFT painful area" and The Back Book, (2) "IFT spinal nerve" and The Back Book, and (3) "Control," The Back Book only. Standardized IFT stimulation parameters were used for 30 minutes' duration. The main outcome measures were; Pain Rating Index, Roland-Morris Disability Questionnaire (RMDQ), and EuroQol were completed by subjects pretreatment, at discharge, and 3-month follow-up. The result was that all groups had significant improvements in all outcomes at follow-up. Subjects managed by IFT spinal nerve and the Back Book displayed both a statistically significant (p = .030) and clinically meaningful reduction in functional disability (RMDQ), compared with management via IFT painful area and the Back Book combined or the Back Book alone. The investigators concluded that the IFT electrode placement technique affects Low Back Pain specific functional disability.

Korom, Mintaze and Yigiter [60] have conducted a study to investigate the effectiveness of Short Wave Diathermy in patients with low back pain. 60

---

[60] Kerem, Mintaze and Yigiter, Effects of Continous and pulsed Short Wave Diathermy in low back pain patients, <u>The Pain Clinic</u>, Vol. 14 (1): 2002: pp 55 – 59.

patients with a diagnosis of disc degeneration and root irritation participated in the study. Patients were divided in to three groups. Each group underwent a different physiotherapy programme. Continuous Short Wave Diathermy and exercises were given to the first group. Pulsed 200 Hz Short Wave Diathermy and exercises were given to the second group, while 46 Hz Pulsed Short Wave Diathermy and exercises were given to the third group. All patients were evaluated for their pain perception level, muscle strength and Lumbar range of motion. Results showed significant improvement in measured parameters in each group after the treatment. However pain relief increase in muscular strength and range of motion were significantly higher in pulsed Short Wave Diathermy group than in those who were treated with continous Short Wave Diathermy. The researchers concluded that all the interventions used in the study were found effective in reducing low back pain, but pulsed Short Wave Diathermy was found to be more effective than continous Short Wave Diathermy.

Nadler, Steiner and Petty [61] have conducted a study to evaluate the efficacy and safety of 8 hours of continuous, low-level heat-wrap therapy administered during sleep, through a prospective, randomized, parallel, single-blind (investigator), placebo-controlled, multicenter clinical trial. The participants were by baseline pain intensity and gender and randomized to one of

---

[61] Nadler.S.F., Steiner.D.J.,and Petty.S.R., Heat-wrap therapy for relief of low back pain, Archives of   Physical   Medicine   and   Rehabilitation, 2003 Mar; 84(3):335-42.

the following treatments: evaluation of efficacy (heatwrap, n=33; oral placebo, n=34) or blinding (unheated wrap, n=5; oral ibuprofen, n=4). All treatments were administered for 3 consecutive nights with 2 days of follow-up. It has been found that Heatwrap therapy was significantly better than placebo at hour 0 on days 2 through 4 for mean pain relief (P=.00005); at hours 0 through 8 on days 2 through 4 for pain relief (P<.001); at hour 0 on day 4 and at hour 0 on day 5 for mean pain relief (P<.001); on day 4 in reduction of morning muscle stiffness (P<.001); for increased lateral trunk flexibility on day 4 (P<.002); and for decreased low back disability on day 4 (P=.005). Adverse events were mild and infrequent. Overnight use of heat-wrap therapy provided effective pain relief throughout the next day, reduced muscle stiffness and disability, and improved trunk flexibility. Positive effects were sustained more than 48 hours after treatments were completed.

Grant et al [62] have studied the efficacy of Transcutaneous electrical nerve stimulation (TENS) on low back pain patients. Sixty patients aged 60 or above, with back pain for at least 6 months were recruited from General Practitioner referrals and randomized to 4 weeks of treatment with Transcutaneous electrical nerve stimulation (TENS) or acupuncture. All treatments were administered by the same physiotherapist and both groups had the same contact with him. The

---

[62] Grant.D.J. et al, Transcutaneous Electrical Nerve Stimulation (TENS) for chronic back pain, Pain, 1999; 82(1): 9-13

following were measured at baseline, completion and at a 3-month follow-up by an independent observer blinded to treatment received: (1) pain severity on visual analogue scale (VAS); (2) pain subscale of Nottingham Health Profile (NHP); (3) number of analgesic tablets consumed in previous week; (4) spinal flexion from C7 to S1. Thirty-two patients were randomized to acupuncture and 28 to TENS; only three withdrew (two from acupuncture, one from TENS). Significant improvements were shown on VAS ($P < 0.001$), NHP ($P < 0.001$) and tablet count ($P < 0.05$) between baseline and completion in both groups, these improvements remaining significant comparing baseline with follow-up with a further non-significant improvement in VAS and NHP in the acupuncture group. The acupuncture but not the TENS patients showed a small but statistically significant improvement ($P < 0.05$) in mean spinal flexion between baseline and completion which was not maintained at follow-up. Thus in these elderly patients with chronic back pain both acupuncture and TENS had demonstrable benefits which out lasted the treatment period.

Khan, Levack and Salih [63] have conducted a study to assess whether Lumbar corsets are effective in reducing low back pain. A postal questionnaire was sent to 130 consecutive patients who had been prescribed lumbar corset for controlling low back pain in two year period. 102 patients (78%) responded. The Greenough and Fraser and Visual analogue scoring system were used to assess

---

[63] Khan.A.M, Levack.B, Salih.M, Lumbar Corset-Effective for low back pain, <u>Hong Kong journal of Orthopeadic Surgery</u>, 2002: 6(1): 34-38

the physical and functional improvement of low back pain. The patients had worn the lumbar corset for more than one year of duration. 90 patients normally worn the corset all day or most part of the day. There was an improvement in the total back pain outcome score before versus after wearing the lumbar corset. It has been found that Greenough and Faser mean; 30.02 up from 20.07 (p<0.0001) and visual analogue mean pain score down to 4.90 from 8.30 (p<0.001). The researchers concluded that lumbar corsets were found effective in reducing low back pain.

Gale and Rothbart [64] have assessed the degree of pain relief obtained by applying infra-red radiation to the low back in patients with chronic, intractable low back pain. 40 patients with chronic low back pain of over 6 years duration were recruited from patients attending a pain management clinic. They were randomly assigned to infra-red radiation therapy or placebo treatment. One patient dropped out of placebo group and as a result 21 patients received infrared radiation and 18 received placebo therapy. Patients attended seven weekly sessions. One baseline and six weekly sets of values were recorded. The principle measure of outcome was pain rated on the numerical rating scale (NRS). It has been found that the mean NRS scores in the treatment group fell from 6.9 of 10 to 3 of 10 at the end of the study. The mean NRS in the placebo

---

[64] Gale.G.D, Rothbart.P.J, Infrared therapy for chronic low back pain, Pain Research Management, 2006 Autumn, 11(3): 193-196

group fell from 7.4 of 10 to 6 of 10. The investigators concluded that infrared radiation therapy was demonstrated to be effective in reducing chronic low back pain and no adverse effects were observed.

Touch Research Institute in conjunction with the University of Miami School of Medicine and Iris Burman of Educating Hands,[65] conducted a study in January 2000 on the effect of Massage therapy on Low back pain. Twenty-four adults who had experienced low-back pain for at least six months were randomly assigned to either a massage therapy group or a relaxation therapy group. The massage therapy group received twice-weekly, 30-minute massages for five weeks. Starting in the prone position, the following techniques were used: kneading and pressing the back muscles, stroking both sides of the spine and hips, gliding strokes to the legs, and kneading and pressing the thighs. Continuing in the supine position, participants received: gliding strokes to the neck and abdomen, kneading of the rectus and oblique muscles that help bend the trunk of the body forward, stroking of the legs, kneading of the anterior thighs, flexing of the thighs and knees, and gentle pulling on both legs. Those in the relaxation group were instructed in progressive muscle relaxation techniques to tense and relax muscles in the feet, calves, thighs, hands, arms, back and face. Participants performed these exercises at home twice weekly for 30 minutes.

---

[65] Hernandez Reif Maria, Field Tiffany, Massage Eases Lower Back Pain, Increases Range of Motion, International Journal of Neuroscience, 2001, Vol. 106, PP.131-145.

Assessments taken before and after the first and last sessions included; the McGill Pain Questionnaire to measure pain; the Visual Analogue Scale to measure present level of pain; the Range of Motion Measures test to rate the level of ability to bend; a Symptom Checklist-90 Revised, to measure moods. Results showed that both groups experienced a decrease in stress and long-term pain, but only the massage group experienced less pain directly after the session, fewer depressive symptoms, improved range of motion. The researchers concluded that the data suggested that massage therapy effectively reduces pain and attenuates psychological symptoms associated with lower back pain.

Walach, Güthlin and König [66] have conducted a study (randomized controlled trial) on classic massage, compared to standard medical care (SMC) in chronic pain conditions of low back. The Outcome measure were; Pain rating (nine-point Likert-scale; predefined main outcome criterion) at pre-treatment, post-treatment, and 3 months follow-up, as well as pain adjective list, depression, anxiety, mood, and body concept. Only 29 patients were randomized, 19 to receive massage, 10 to SMC. Pain decreased significantly in both groups, but only in the massage group, it still significantly decreased at follow-up. Depression and anxiety were also decreased significantly by both treatments, yet only in the massage group maintained at follow up. The

---

[66] Harald Walach, Corina Guthlin, Miriam Konig, Efficacy of Massage Therapy in Chronic low back Pain, The Journal of Alternative and Complementary Medicine, 2003, 9(6): 837-846.

researchers concluded that despite its limitation resulting from problems with numbers and randomization the study shows that massage can be at least as effective as SMC in chronic low back pain syndromes .

Battie, Cherkin and Dunn [67] have studied the effectiveness of McKenzie method in the treatment of low back pain. Low Back pain was estimated to account for 45% of patient visits to physical therapists. The researchers concluded that McKenzie method which is mostly based on specific exercises, corretion of posture, education to the patient and prophylaxis of recurrence of symptoms with self treatment was deemed the most useful approach for managing patients with low back pain, especially of mechanical origin and education in body mechanics, stretching, strengthening exercises, and aerobic exercises were among the most common treatment preferences.

Cherkin, Eisenberg and Sherman,[68] have studied the effectiveness of therapeutic massage, acupuncture and self-care education for persistent low back pain. They randomized 262 patients aged 20 to 70 years who had persistent low back pain to receive Traditional Chinese Medical acupuncture (n = 94), therapeutic massage (n = 78), or self-care educational materials (n = 90). Up to

---

[67] Battie.M.C., Cherkin.D.C., Dunn.R., Efficacy of McKenzie Method for treating Low back pain, <u>Physical Therapy</u>, Vol. 74, No. 3, March 1994, PP.219-226

[68] Daniel.C.Cherkin, David Eisenberg, Karen.J.Sherman, Therapeutic Massage, Chinese Medical Acupuncture, and Self-care Education for Chronic Low Back Pain <u>Archieves of Internal Medicine</u>, 2001; 161(8):1081-1088.

10 massage or acupuncture visits were permitted over 10 weeks. Symptoms (0-10 scale) and dysfunction (0-23 scale) were assessed by telephone interviewers masked to treatment group. Follow-up was available for 95% of patients after 4, 10, and 52 weeks, and none withdrew for adverse effects. Treatment groups were compared after adjustment for pre-randomization covariates using an intent-to-treat analysis. At 10 weeks, massage was superior to self-care on the symptom scale (3.41 vs 4.71, respectively; $P = .01$) and the disability scale (5.88 vs 8.92, respectively; $P<.001$). Massage was also superior to acupuncture on the disability scale (5.89 vs 8.25, respectively; $P = .01$). After 1 year, massage was not better than self-care but was better than acupuncture (symptom scale: 3.08 vs 4.74, respectively; $P = .002$; dysfunction scale: 6.29 vs 8.21, respectively; $P = .05$). The massage group used the least medications ($P<.05$) and had the lowest costs of subsequent care. Researchers concluded that Therapeutic massage was effective for persistent low back pain, apparently providing long-lasting benefits. Traditional Chinese Medical acupuncture was relatively ineffective. Massage might be an effective alternative to conventional medical care for persistent low back pain.

Chok et al[69] have conducted research in order to evaluate the effectiveness of trunk extensor endurance training in reducing pain and

---

[69] Beverley Chok, Seang Beng Tan, Raymond Lee, Jane Latimer; Endurance Training of the Trunk Extensor Muscles in People with Subacute Low Back Pain, <u>Physical Therapy</u>, Vol. 79, No. 11, November 1999, PP. 1032 1042

decreasing disability in subjects with subacute low back pain (ie, onset of back pain within 7 days to 7 weeks). Patients were randomly assigned to either an experimental group or a control group. A visual analog scale and the Pain Rating Index (PRI) of the McGill Pain Questionnaire (MPQ) were used to obtain baseline measurements of pain. The Roland-Morris Disability Questionnaire (RMDQ) was used to measure disability, and the Sorensen Test was used to measure trunk extensor endurance. Subjects in the experimental group attended exercise sessions 3 times per week for 6 weeks. Subjects in the control group did not do exercises. Both groups were given back care advice and hot packs for 15 minutes, 3 to 5 times per week. Reassessments were carried out at 3 and 6 weeks.

It has been found that there were differences between the 2 groups at 3 weeks with regard to pain intensity during the evaluation session, pain experienced over the preceding 24 hours, the total MPQ PRI, the sensory component of the MPQ PRI, and the RMDQ. At 6 weeks, no differences were found for pain measurements, disability scores, and holding time on the Sorensen Test. The researchers concluded that the trunk extensor endurance training reduced pain and improved function at 3 weeks period but resulted in no improvement at 6 weeks period, when compared with the control group. Endurance exercise is considered to expedite the recovery process for patients with an acute episode of low back pain.

Chatzitheodorou and Kabitsis,[70] have studied the effects of high-intensity aerobic exercise on pain, disability and psychological strain, in people with chronic low back pain. Twenty subjects receiving primary health care were randomly allocated in to exercise and control groups. Subjects in the exercise group received a 12-week, high-intensity aerobic exercise program. Subjects in the control group received 12 weeks of passive modalities without any form of physical activity. Data analysis identified reductions in pain (41%, t_{10}=8.51, P<.001), disability (31%, t_{10}=7.32, P<.001), and psychological strain (35%, t_{10}=7.09, P<.001) in subjects in the exercise group and no changes in subjects in the control group. The investigators concluded that regular high-intensity aerobic exercise alleviated pain, disability, and psychological strain in subjects with chronic low back pain.

A study conducted by O'Sullivan et al [71] on the evaluation of Specific Stabilizing Exercises in the treatment of Chronic Low Back Pain with Radiologic diagnosis of Spondylolysis or Spondylolisthesis, in which forty four patients with this condition were assigned randomly into two treatment groups. The first group underwent a 10-week specific exercise treatment programme involving the specific training of the deep abdominal muscles, with co-activation

---

[70] Dimitris Chatzitheodorou, Chris Kabitsis, Effects of High-Intensity Aerobic Exercise and Chronic Low Back Pain, Physical Therapy, Vol. 87, No. 3, March 2007, PP. 304-312

[71] O'Sullivan et al, Evaluation of Specific Stabilizing Exercises in the treatment of Chronic Low Book Pain, Spine, 1997 Dec 15, 22(24):2959-2967.

of the lumbar multifidus proximal to the pars defects. The activation of these muscles was incorporated into previously aggravating static postures and functional tasks. The control group underwent treatment as directed by their treating practitioner. After the experiment, the specific exercise group showed a statistically significant reduction in pain intensity and functional disability levels, which means that a "specific exercise" treatment approach appears more effective than other commonly prescribed conservative treatment programmes in patients with chronically symptomatic spondylolysis or spondylolisthesis.

Norfolk [72] has done a comparative study between the range of lumbar movement of two groups of people of comparable age under the influence of Williams' exercises which was designed to improve the flexibility of the lower back and to correct the common tendency to over extend the lumbar spine. This exclude backward-bending exercises simply because these movements may often aggravate back troubles. Carrying out these exercises regularly will secure a marked improvement in spinal flexibility within a month. This has been proved by trials carried out at the University of Taxas Health Science Center, Dallas. Out of the two study groups, the first group had low back pain and the second group had nothing. Measurements showed that the patients complaining of pain were invariably stiffer than their partners who were pain free. On average, the patients could manage no more than 37°of lumbar movement, whereas the

---

[72] Donald Norfolk, <u>Conquering Back Pain,</u> Blandford Press, London, 1997, PP.70-72.

control group could swing their lumbar spines through an arc of 82°. To overcome this handicap the patients were instructed to perform "Williams' exercises" three times a day. On testing after a period of three weeks, they showed an avearge range of 65° of lumbar movement, a remarkable increase in spinal flexibility of 72 pecent.

Hayden et al [73] have studied the effectiveness of exercise therapy in adult nonspecific acute, sub-acute, and chronic low back pain versus no treatment and other conservative treatments. Study selection was randomized, controlled trials evaluating exercise therapy for adult nonspecific low back pain and measuring pain, function, rcturn to work or absenteeism, and global improvement outcomes. Two reviewers independently selected studies and extracted data on study characteristics, quality, and outcomes at short-, intermediate-, and long-term follow-up. 61 randomized, controlled trials (6390 participants) met inclusion criteria: acute (11 trials), subacute (6 trials), and chronic (43 trials) low back pain (1 trial was unclear). Evidence suggested that exercise therapy is effective in chronic back pain relative to comparisons at all follow-up periods. Pooled mean improvement (of 100 points) was 7.3 points (95% CI, 3.7 to 10.9 points) for pain and 2.5 points (CI, 1.0 to 3.9 points) for function at earliest follow-up. In studies investigating patients (people seeking care for back pain), mean improvement

---

[73] Jill A Hayden et al , Exercise Therapy for Nonspecific Low Back Pain-A Meta Analysis, Annals of Internal Medicine, 3 May 2005, Volume 142, Issue 9, Pages 765-775

was 13.3 points (CI, 5.5 to 21.1 points) for pain and 6.9 points (CI, 2.2 to 11.7 points) for function, compared with studies where some participants had been recruited from a general population (for example, with advertisements). Some evidence suggested effectiveness of a graded-activity exercise program in sub-acute low back pain in occupational settings, although the evidence for other types of exercise therapy in other populations is inconsistent. In acute low back pain, exercise therapy and other programs were equally effective (pain, 0.03 point [CI, −1.3 to 1.4 points]). Exercise therapy seems to be slightly effective at decreasing pain and improving function in adults with chronic low back pain, particularly in health care populations. In sub-acute low back pain populations, some evidence suggested that a graded-activity program improves absenteeism outcomes, although evidence for other types of exercise is unclear. In acute low back pain populations, exercise therapy is as effective as either no treatment or other conservative treatments.

Tulder, Koes and Bouter[74] have conducted a study to assess the effectiveness of the most common conservative types of treatment for patients with acute and chronic non specific low back pain. A rating system was used to assess the strength of the evidence, based on the methodologic quality of the randomized controlled trials, the relevance of outcome measures and the consistency of results. The number of randomized controlled trials identified

---

[74] Van Tulder.M.W., Koes.B.W., Bouter.L.M, Conservative treatment of acute and chronic non specific low back pain, <u>ACP Journal Club,</u> 1998 May-Jun;128(3):65.

varied widely with regard to the interventions involved. Strong evidence was found for the effectiveness of muscle relaxants and non-steroidal anti-inflammatory drugs for acute low back pain. Strong evidence also was found for the effectiveness of manipulation, back schools, and exercise therapy for chronic low back pain, especially for short term effects.

Malmivaara, Häkkinen and Aro[75] have studied the impact of bed rest and back-extension exercises which are often prescribed for patients with acute low back pain, but the effectiveness of which remains controversial. They conducted a controlled trial among employees of the city of Helsinki, Finland, who presented to an occupational health care center with acute, nonspecific low back pain. The patients were randomly assigned to one of three treatments; bed rest for two days (67 patients), back-mobilizing exercises (52 patients), or the continuation of ordinary activities as tolerated (the control group; 67 patients). Outcomes were assessed after 3 and 12 weeks. After 3 and 12 weeks, the patients in the control group had better recovery than those prescribed either bed rest or exercises. There were statistically significant differences favouring the control group in the duration of pain, pain intensity, lumbar flexion, ability to work as measured subjectively, Oswestry back-disability index, and number of days absent from work. Recovery was slowest among the patients assigned to bed

---

[75] Antti Malmivaara, Unto Häkkinen, Timo Aro, The Treatment of Acute Low Back Pain - Bed Rest, Exercise or Ordinary Activity, The New England journal of Medicine, Volume: 332:351-355, Feb. 9, 1995, No.6

rest. Among patients with acute low back pain, continuing ordinary activities within the limits permitted by the pain led to more rapid recovery than either bed rest or back-mobilizing exercises.

Ongley et al [76] have conducted a study in which 81 patients with chronic low back pain (average duration 10 years) were randomised to two treatment groups. 40 received an empirically devised regimen of forceful spinal manipulation and injections of a dextrose-glycerine-phenol ("proliferant") solution into soft-tissue structures, as part of a programme to decrease pain and disability. The other 41 patients received parallel treatment in which the main differences were less extensive initial local anaesthesia and manipulation, and substitution of saline for proliferant. Neither patients nor assessors knew which treatment had been given. When assessed by disability scores, the experimental group had greater improvement than the control group at one (p less than 0.001), three (p less than 0.004), and six (p less than 0.001) months from the end of treatment; at six months an improvement of more than 50% was recorded in 35 of the experimental group versus 16 of the control group and the numbers free from disability were 15 and 4, respectively (p less than 0.003). Visual analogue pain scores and pain diagrams likewise showed significant advantages for the experimental regimen.

---

[76] Ongley.M.J, Klein.R.G., Dorman.T.A., Eek.B.C., Hubert.L.J., A new approach to the treatment of chronic low back pain, Lancet Journal, 1987 Jul. 18;2(8551):143-46.

Moseley [77] has conducted a study to determine the efficacy of a combined physiotherapy treatment that comprised strategies like; Manual therapy, exercise and education. By concealed randomisation, 57 chronic low back pain patients were allocated to either the four-week physiotherapy program or management as directed by their general practitioners. The dependent variables of interest were pain and disability. Assessors were blind to treatment group. Outcome data from 49 subjects (86%) showed a significant treatment effect. The physiotherapy program reduced pain and disability by a mean of 1.5/10 points on a numerical rating scale (95% CI 0.7 to 2.3) and 3.9 points on the 18-point Roland Morris Disability Questionnaire (95% CI 2 to 5.8), respectively. The number needed to treat in order to gain a clinically meaningful change was 3 (95% CI 3 to 8) for pain, and 2 (95% CI 2 to 5) for disability. A treatment effect was maintained at one-year follow-up. The findings supported the efficacy of combined physiotherapy treatment in producing symptomatic and functional change in moderately disabled chronic low back pain patients.

Pengel et al[78], have investigated the effectiveness of physiotherapist-prescribed exercise, advice, or both for subacute low back pain through a Factorial randomized, placebo-controlled trial. As experiment centers, 7

---

[77] Moseley L., Combined Physiotherapy and Education is efficacious for chronic low back pain, Australian Journal of Physiotherapy, 2002; 48(4):297-302.

[78] Pengel,L.H et al, Physiotherapist-directed exercise, advice, or both for sub-acute low back pain, Annals of Internal Medicine; 2007 Jun. 5;146(11):787-96

university hospitals and primary care clinics in Australia and New Zealand were chosen. The patients were 259 persons with subacute low back pain (>6 weeks and <3 months in duration). The Participants were given 12 physiotherapist-directed exercise or sham exercise sessions and 3 physiotherapist-directed advice or sham advice sessions over 6 weeks. Primary outcomes were average pain over the past week (scale, 0 to 10), function (Patient-Specific Functional Scale), and global perceived effect (11-point scale) at 6 weeks and 12 months. Secondary outcomes were disability (Roland-Morris Disability Questionnaire), number of health care contacts, and depression (Depression Anxiety Stress Scales-21). It has been found that Exercise and advice were each slightly more effective than placebo at 6 weeks but not at 12 months. The effect of advice on the pain scale was -0.7 point (95% CI, -1.2 to -0.2 point; P = 0.011) at 6 weeks and -0.4 point (CI, -1.0 to 0.3 point; P = 0.27) at 12 months, whereas the effect of exercise was -0.8 point (CI, -1.3 to -0.3 point; P = 0.004) at 6 weeks and -0.5 point (CI, -1.1 to 0.2 point; P = 0.14) at 12 months. The effect of advice on the function scale was 0.7 point (CI, 0.1 to 1.3 points; P = 0.014) at 6 weeks and 0.6 point (CI, 0.1 to 1.2 points; P = 0.023) at 12 months, and the effect of exercise was 0.4 point (CI, -0.2 to 1.0 point; P = 0.174) at 6 weeks and 0.5 point (CI, -0.1 to 1.0 point; P = 0.094) at 12 months. The effect of advice on the global perceived effect scale was 0.8 point (CI, 0.3 to 1.2 points; P < 0.001) at 6 weeks and 0.3 point (CI, -0.2 to 0.9 point; P = 0.24) at 12 months, and the effect of exercise was 0.5 point (CI, 0.1 to 1.0 point; P = 0.017) at 6 weeks and 0.4 point (CI, -0.1 to 1.0 point; P = 0.134) at 12 months. When administered together, exercise and advice had larger effects on all outcomes at 6 weeks (effect on pain, -1.5 [CI -2.2 to -0.7 point; P = 0.001], with similar results for other primary outcomes); however, by 12 months, there was a statistically significant effect only for function (effect, 1.1 points [CI, 0.3 to 1.8 points]; P = 0.005). The investigators concluded that in participants with subacute low back pain, physiotherapist-directed exercise and advice were each slightly more effective than placebo at 6 weeks.

Snook et al, [79] have conducted a study to test the hypothesis that the control of lumbar flexion in the early morning will significantly reduce chronic, nonspecific low back pain. Previous studies have indicated an increased risk of low back pain with bending forward in the early morning, primarily because of increased fluid content in the intervertebral discs at that time. After 6 months of recording baseline data, 85 subjects with persistent or recurring low back pain were randomly assigned to treatment and control groups. The treatment group received instruction in the control of early morning lumbar flexion. The control group received a sham treatment of six exercises shown to be ineffective in reducing low back pain. Six months later, the control group received the experimental treatment, Diaries were used to record daily levels of pain intensity, disability, impairment, and medication usage. Significant reductions in pain intensity (P < 0.01) were recorded for the treatment group, but not for the control group (point estimate, 33%; 95% confidence interval, 11-55%). After

---

[79] Snook,S.H. et al, Early morning Lumbar flexion, Spine 1998, Dec. 1;23(23):2601-07.

receiving the experimental treatment, the control group responded with similar reductions ($P < 0.05$). Significant reductions also were observed in total days in pain, disability, impairment, and medication usage. The conclusion was; controlling lumbar flexion in the early morning is a form of self-care with potential for reducing chronic, nonspecific low back pain.

Erhard, Delitto and Cibulka [80] have examined the relative effectiveness of an extension programme and a manipulation program with flexion and extension exercises in patients with low back syndrome. Forty nine patients with less than a 3 months history of low back pain were seen at physical therapy clinics in western Pennsylvania, southern Mississippi, and eastern Missouri during a 6 months period. Twenty seven of the 49 patients were classified a priori into a treatment-oriented category of extension/ mobilization and were then randomly assigned to participate in an extension program or a program of manipulation followed by hand-heel rocks (flexion and extension). Three patients dropped out of the study for some reasons. The remaining 24 patients (15 male, 9 female; mean age = 44 years, SD = 15, range = 14-73) were assigned randomly and equally to the two groups. Eight physical therapists participated in the study. A randomized clinical trial comparing the two regimens was conducted for a 1-

---

[80] Erhard.R.E., Delitto.A., Cibulka.M.T., Relative effectiveness of an Extension program and a combined program of Manipulation and Flexion and Extension exercises in patients with acute low back syndrome, Physical Therapy, Vol.74, No.12, December 1994, PP.1093-1100

week period. Outcome was assessed using an Oswestry Low Back Pain Questionnaire initially (before treatment) and at 3 and 5 days post-treatment, and data were analyzed using a 2 x 3 (group x time) analysis of variance. A significant interaction of the group and time variables was demonstrated, indicating that the rate of positive response was greater in the manipulation/ hand-heel rock group than in the extension group. It has been found that in the category of patients with low back pain, the use of manipulation as an adjunct to an ongoing exercise program appears to be warranted.

Hoehler, Tobis and Buerger [81] have conducted a randomized clinical trial of rotational manipulation on 95 patients with low back pain selected for (1) the absence of any contra-indications for vertebral manipulation, (2) the absence of any psycho-social problems that might affect the outcome of treatment, (3) the absence of any previous experience with manipulative therapy, and (4) the presence of palpatory cues indicating that manipulation might be successful. Patients were randomly assigned to one of two groups: an experimental group receiving manipulation therapy and a control group receiving soft-tissue massage. Comparison of the two groups indicated that (1) patients who received manipulative treatment were much more likely to report immediate relief after the first treatment, and (2) at discharge, there was no significant difference between the two groups because both showed substantial improvement.

---

[81] K.Hoehler.F.K., Tobis.J.S., Buerger.A.A., Spinal Manipulation for low back pain, <u>JAMA, (The Journal of the American Medical Association)</u>, Vol.245, No.18, May 8,1981.

Aure, Nilsen and Vasseljen [82] have compared the effect of manual therapy to exercise therapy in sick-listed patients with chronic low back pain (>8 wks). In this study, Patients with chronic low back pain or radicular pain sick-listed for more than 8 weeks and less than 6 months were included. A total of 49 patients were randomized to either manual therapy (n = 27) or to exercise therapy (n = 22). Sixteen treatments were given over the course of 2 months. Pain intensity, functional disability (Oswestry disability index), general health (Dartmouth COOP function charts), and return to work were recorded before, immediately after, at 4 weeks, 6 months, and 12 months after the treatment period. Spinal range of motion (Schober's test) was measured before and immediately after the treatment period. Although significant improvements were observed in both groups, the manual therapy group showed significantly larger improvements than the exercise therapy group on all outcome variables throughout the entire experimental period. Immediately after the 2-month treatment period, 67% in the manual therapy and 27% in the exercise therapy group had returned to work (P < 0.01), a relative difference that was maintained throughout the follow-up period. The researchers concluded that improvements were found in both intervention groups, but manual therapy showed significantly greater improvement than exercise therapy in patients with chronic low back pain. The effects were reflected on all outcome measures, both on short and long-term follow-up.

---

[82] Aure.O.F, Nilsen. J.H., Vasseljen.O; Manual therapy and Exercise therapy in patients with chronic low back pain:., Spine, 2003 Mar.15;28(6): 525-531.

Hemmila,[83] has investigated the effects of various therapies in patients with chronic back pain. Chronic back pain has mainly been highlighted only in a relatively small proportion of patients whose conditions require high-cost treatment and present a significant burden on healthcare resources. There has been little evaluation of patients' choices of therapy, particularly alternative/ complementary therapies. Study subjects were 114 Finnish patients, being treated by their General Practitioners for chronic low back pain. They were studied for 1 year before and for 1 year after they entered a randomized clinical trial. Data were obtained from the Social Insurance Institution files, patients' records and questionnaires (the Nottingham Health Profile; NHP) on therapy use, effects of physiotherapy, bone setting and light exercise therapy on these measures were also explored. 1 year before they entered the clinical trial, a third of patients, had consulted their GPs. 50% of the patients had undergone some form of therapy, the main ones being massage, physiotherapy, naprapathy or bone setting. Physiotherapy and bone setting both resulted in improvements on more subscales on the NHP in comparison with exercise. It has been concluded that the quality of life of patients with chronic back pain seemed to be improved by Physiotherapy and bone setting.

---

[83] Hemmila.H.M., Quality of life and care of Back Pain Patients in Finnish general-practice, Spine-27(6):647-653, March-2002.

Delitto, Cibulka and Erhard [84] have conducted a study on the prescriptive validity of a treatment-oriented extension-mobilization category for patients with low back syndrome (LBS). Of a total of 39 patients with LBS referred for physical therapy, 24 patients (14 male, 10 female), aged 14 to 50 years (means = 31.3, SD = 11.6), were classified as having signs and symptoms indicating treatment with an extension-mobilization approach. The remaining subjects were dismissed from the study. Patients in the extension-mobilization category were randomly assigned to either an experimental (treatment) group (n = 14) or a comparison group (n = 10). The experimental and comparison group subjects were treated with either mobilization and extension (a treatment matched to the category) or a flexion exercise regimen (an unmatched treatment). Outcome was assessed with a modified Oswestry Low Back Pain Questionnaire administered initially and at 3 and 5 days after initiation of treatment. Data were analyzed with a 2 x 3 (treatment group x treatment period) analysis of variance. The subjects' rate of improvement, as indicated by the Oswestry questionnaire scores, was dependent on the treatment group to which they were assigned. Subjects treated with extension and mobilization positively responded at a faster rate than did those treated with a flexion-oriented program.

---

[84] Delitto.A., Cibulka.M.T., Erhard.R.E., Extension-Mobilization for acute low back syndrome, Physical Therapy :Vol. 73, No. 4, April 1993, PP.216-222

Cherkin and Sherman[85] have studied about the effectiveness of the popular complementary and alternative medical therapies used to treat low back pain. Systematic reviews of randomized, controlled trials (RCTs) that were published since 1995 and that evaluated massage therapy, or spinal manipulation for nonspecific back pain and RCTs published since the reviews were conducted. Two authors independently extracted data from the reviews (including number of RCTs, type of back pain, quality assessment, and conclusions) and original articles (including type of pain, comparison treatments, sample size, outcomes, follow-up intervals, loss to follow-up, and authors' conclusions). The three RCTs that evaluated massage reported that this therapy is effective for subacute and chronic low back pain. A meta-regression analysis of the results of 26 RCTs evaluating spinal manipulation for acute and chronic low back pain reported that spinal manipulation was superior to sham therapies and therapies judged to have no evidence of a benefit but was not superior to effective conventional treatments. Initial studies have found massage to be effective for persistent low back pain. Spinal manipulation has small clinical benefits that are equivalent to those of other commonly used therapies.

---

[85] Cherkin D.C, Sherman.K.J., Effectiveness of Massage therapy and Spinal manipulation for low back pain., <u>Annals of Internal Medicine</u>, 2003:June 3;138(11):898-906.

Mohseni-Bandpei, Critchley and Staunton [86] have conducted a study to assess the short- and long-term effectiveness of spinal manipulation therapy, and to identify the effect of manipulation on lumbar muscle endurance in patients with chronic low back pain. One hundred and twenty patients with chronic Low back pain were allocated at random into the manipulation/ exercise group or the ultrasound/ exercise group. Both groups were given a programme of exercises. In addition, one group received spinal manipulation therapy and the other group received therapeutic ultrasound. Pain intensity, functional disability, lumbar movements and muscle endurance were measured shortly before treatment, at the end of the treatment programme and 6 months after randomisation using surface electromyography.

Following the treatment, the manipulation/exercise group showed a statistically significant improvement ($P = 0.001$) in pain intensity [mean 16.4 mm, 95% confidence interval (CI) 6.1–26.8], functional disability (mean 8%, 95% CI 2–13) and spinal mobility (flexion: mean 9.4 mm, 95% CI 5.5–13.4; extension: mean 3.4 mm, 95% CI 1.0–5.8). There was no significant difference ($P = 0.068$) between the two groups in the median frequency of surface electromyography (multifidus: mean 6.8 Hz, 95% CI 1.24–14.91; iliocostalis:

---

[86] Mohammad.A.Mohseni-Bandpei, Jacqueline Critchley, Thomas Staunton, Effectiveness of Spinal manipulation therapy and Ultra sound therapy in patients with chronic low back pain, Physical Therapy Vol:92; Issue 1; March 2006; PP.34-42

mean 2.4 Hz, 95% CI 2.5–7.1), although a significant difference ($P = 0.013$) was found in the median frequency slope of surface electromyography in favour of spinal manipulation for multifidus alone (mean 0.3, 95% CI 0.1–0.5). A significant difference was also found between the two groups in favour of the manipulation/exercise group at 6-month follow-up. The reseachers concluded that although improvements were recorded in both groups, patients receiving manipulation/ exercise showed a greater improvement compared with those received ultra sound/ exercise at both the end of the treatment period and at 6-month follow-up.

Fox and Melzack[87] have conducted research on the effect of Transcutaneous electrical nerve stimulation and acupuncture on low back pain patients. Twelve patients suffering chronic low-back pain were treated with both acupuncture and Transcutaneous electrical stimulation. The order of treatments was balanced, and changes in the intensity and quality of pain were measured with the McGill Pain Questionnaire. The results, based on a measure of overall pain intensity, showed that pain relief greater than 33% was produced in 75% of the patients by acupuncture and in 66% by Transcutanious electrical stimulation. The mean duration of pain relief was 40 hrs after acupuncture and 23 hrs after electrical stimulation. Although the mean scores are larger for acupuncture than

---

[87] Elisabeth.J.Fox, Ronald Melzack, Transcutaneous Electrical nerve stimulation (TENS) and Acupuncture, Comparison of treatments for low-back pain, Pain, Volume 2, Issue 2, June 1976, PP.141-148.

for transcutaneous electrical stimulation, statistical analysis of the data failed to reveal significant differences between the two treatments on any of the measures. Both methods, therefore, appear to be equally effective, and probably have the same underlying mechanism of action. Consideration of the advantages and disadvantages of the two methods suggests that Transcutaneous electrical stimulation is potentially the more practical, since it can be administered under supervision by paramedical personnel.

Clark and Sterner[88] have conducted a study (randomized controlled trial) with regard to the effect of therapeutic Ultra-sound treatment on low back pain patients and concluded that ultra sound reduced spasm in lumbar radiculopathy. It has also been found that an ultra sound treatment varying from 8 to 10 minutes is ideal for acute Low back pain. The investigators studied 40 patients consulting their general practitioners for low back pain, who have been treated with ultra sound therapy (20 patients) and with sham treatment procedure (20 patients). Main outcome measure was scores on the Roland Morris disability questionnaire at the baseline and after 2 months. After the treatment period, Ultra sound group showed statistically significant improvement, when compared to sham treatment group. Also no serious adverse events have been noticed as result of the treatment.

---

[88] Clark.GR, Sterner.L, Use of Therapeutic Ultra Sound, <u>Physiotherapy,</u> 1976, 62 (185)

2.5 SUMMERISATION OF THE REVIEW

The above studies have vehemently shown that Yoga, Naturopthy and Physiotherapy have positive effect on low back pain patients. From the thirteen studies described and nineteen studies mentioned with regard to the administration of Yogic practices, it has been revealed that low back pain has been reduced considerably by Yogic practices. From the seven studies described and the other seven studies mentioned with regard to the administration of Naturopathic treatment, it has been revealed that Naturopathic treatment was very effective on low back pain patients. From the thirtyone studies described with regard to the administration of Physiotherapy treatment on low back pain patients, it has been proved that there is positive effect for Physiotherapy treatment on low back pain patients.

Chapter iii

METHODOLOGY

Chapter iii

METHODOLOGY

3.1 INTRODUCTION

The methodology of the study endeavours an overview of all the considerations of the research work that is to be executed and at this stage, the crucial decisions for the accomplishment of the objectives of the study, are taken.

According to Kothari [1], Research Methodology is a way to systematically solve the problem of the "Research".

It is the science of method, the science dealing with principles of procedure in research and study.[2] It is a science that deals with the various steps, which are generally adopted by a research scholar in studying his research problem along with the logic behind it. In fact the successful completion of a research work requires proper planning. The planning includes; various measures to be adopted for the collection of relevant data, the sample to be taken, the controls to be employed and which would be the pertinent data.

---

[1] Kothari.C.R., <u>Research Methodology – Methods and Techniques</u>, Vishwaprakashan Publishers, New Delhi, 1996

[2] <u>Dorlands' Medical Dictionary for Health Consumer</u>, W.B.Saunders, Philadelphia, 2007

be taken, the controls to be employed and which would be the pertinent data, that would be analysed. The details regarding the methods adopted, tools and techniques used, samples selected, procedure adopted and statistical techniques employed are given in this chapter.

3.2 SELECTION OF SUBJECTS

One Hundred low back pain patients, (73 males & 27 females) aged between 30 and 60 years of age had been taken for the study. The subjects were all low back pain patients, out of which 53 patients were afflicted with low back pain alone and 47 were with low back pain and leg pain. Among the subjects, 86 had taken some treatments earlier. In the case of low back pain, the maximum duration of pain was 1 year & 8 months and the minimum duration of pain was 3 months. In the case of, leg pain the maximum duration of pain was 1 year 6 months and the minimum duration was $2\frac{1}{2}$ months. The subjects were divided into five groups; namely Yoga group, Naturopathy group, Physiotherapy group,Yoga and Naturopathy group and Control group. Each group comprised 20 subjects. Among the subjects, there were Office staff (19 nos.), Drivers (9 nos.), House wives (9 nos.), School/College teachers (12nos.), Sales executives (5nos.), Company/Factory workers (10 nos.), Computer Operators (8 nos.) Business Men/Shop Keepers (7 nos.), Sales Assistants (5 nos.), Security Guards (3 nos.), Loading workers (4 nos.), Bank Staff (6 nos.) and Journalist/Insurance Adviser/Hotel Bearer (1 no.each). There were also people who had been suffering from low back pain as a result of minor accidents.

3.3 SELECTION OF VARIABLES IN THE EXPERIMENT

Variables are the characteristics or conditions that are manipulated , controlled and observed by the Investigator. For this study, the investigator reviewed the available scientific literature pertaining to the effects of Yogic practices, Naturopathy and Physiotherapy on low back pain patients from books, journals/ periodicals, web sites and research papers. Taking into consideration of the relevance to the study and the feasibility criteria, the following variables have been selected for this study, which are broadly classified as; Independent variables and Dependent variables.

Independent Variables

In this study, the independent variables are Yoga (Group I), Naturopathy (Group II), Physiotherapy (Group III) and Yoga & Naturopathy (Group IV) .

Dependent Variables

Here the dependent variables are pain intensity, personal care (washing, dressing etc). lifting, walking, sitting. standing, sleeping, social life, travelling. employment/home making, Disability index (total), Quadruple visual analogue scale , Spinal flexion and low back pain.

3.4 EXPERIMENTAL DESIGN

Participants (twenty each) were randomly assigned to either Yoga group, Naturopathy group, Physiotherapy group, Combined Yoga and Naturopathy group or Control group. The experiment was for a period of 12 weeks. All the participants who enrolled in the study have completed the study. Participants reported on a variety of outcomes at baseline and at the end of the 12 weeks intervention.

3.5 TOOLS / TECHNIQUES USED

Keeping in view of the objectives of the study, the following tools and techniques were used.

In the Pre-test and in the Post-test, Low back pain has been assessed by using the Oswestry disability questionnaire. The questionnaire was specifically intented for collecting the data before and after the experiments/ treatments. The questionnaire was designed by the Department of Spinal Disorders, Robert Jones and Agnes Hunt Orthopaedic Hospital, Oswestry, Shropshire, UK and the same is given in Appendix – i. This questionnaire had been designed to give the investigator, information as to how the patient's low back pain has affected his/her ability to manage in everyday life. The Oswestry disability index is an extremely important tool that researchers and disability evaluators use to measure a patient's permenant functional disability. The test is considered as the "gold standard" of low back functional outcome tools. In the questionnaire, there are ten sections such as Pain intensity. Personal care (dressing/washing), Lifting, Walking, Sitting, Standing, Sleeping, Social life, Travelling, Employment/ Home making. There are six statements for each section. The score pattern is; for statement no.1, the score is 0 and for statement no.2, the score is 1 and for statement no.6, the score is 5. To find out the disability index (total- percentage), add up the points and then divide this number by 50, then multiply it by 100.

Low Back pain has also been assessed in the pre-test and in the post-test by modified Schober's test. Here the range of Spinal flexion was measured. When the spine flexes, the distance between successive vertebral spines increases. By measuring the spine when the patient is errect, and then when bend forwards, any gain gives unequivocal evidence of spinal flexion. The practice accepted internationally (originated from U.K.) is to employ a 15 cm length of spine.(which has been shown to give the most reliable results). Begin by positioning a tape measure by with the 10 cm mark level with the dimples of Venus. (which mark the posterior superior iliac spines). Mark the skin at the end of the tape, ie; at zero and also at 15 cm. Then anchor the top of the tape with a finger and ask the patient to flex as far forward as he/she can. Note where the 15 cm mark strikes the tape and work out the increment, which is entirely due to lumbar spine flexion.

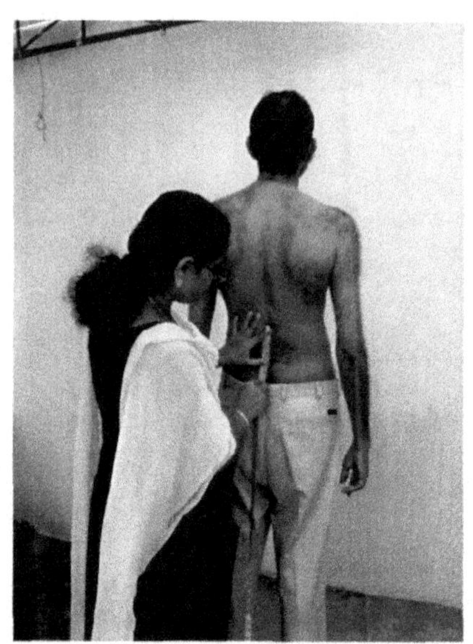

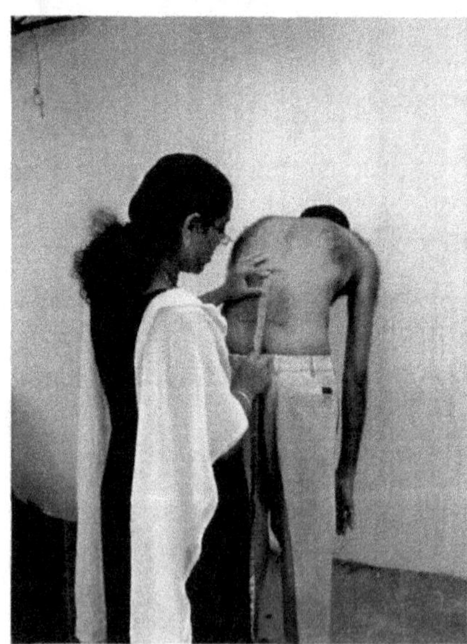

The Investigator measures Spinal Flexion of the Subject (Schober's Test)

The Quadruple Visual Analogue Scale also has been used to assess the pain level of the patients before and after the experiment. The Visual Analogue Scale (VAS) is a measurement instrument to measure a characteristic or attitude that is believed to range across a continuum of values and can't easily be directlty measured. For eg. The amount of pain that a patient feels ranges across a continuum from none to an extreme amount of pain. From the patient's perspective this spectrum appears continuous, ie; their pain does not take discrete jumps, as a categorization of none, mild, moderate and severe would suggest. It was to capture this idea of an underlying continuum that the Visual Analogue Scale was devised.

Operationally the VAS is usually a horizondal line, 100 mm in length, anchored by word descriptors at each end (as illustrated below). The patient marks on the line the point that they feel represents their perception of their current state. The VAS score is determined by measuring in millimeters from the left hand end of the line to the point that the patient marks. As such the assessment is clearly highly subjective, these scales are of most value when looking at change within individuals.

Quadruple Visual Analogue Scale

Patient Name ____

Date ___________________________________

(**Instructions:** Please circle the number that best describes the question being asked.
Note:- Please indicate your low back pain level right now, average pain, and pain at its best and worst.)

1 – What is your pain RIGHT NOW?

No pain   0   1   2   3   4   5   6   7   8   9   10   **worst possible**

2 – What is your TYPICAL or AVERAGE pain?

No pain   0   1   2   3   4   5   6   7   8   9   10   **worst possible**

3 – What is your pain level AT ITS BEST (How close to "0" does your pain get at its best)?

No pain   0   1   2   3   4   5   6   7   8   9   10   **worst possible**

4 – What is your pain level AT ITS WORST (How close to "10" does your pain get at its worst)?

No pain   0   1   2   3   4   5   6   7   8   9   10   **worst possible**

OTHER COMMENTS:

____

____

Examiner

Here the first question is about the pain level at the time of the current patient visit. The second question is about the typical or average pain. since the last visit. (or since the onset of the condition-depending on the chronocity of the condition). The third question is about the pain level at it's best, since the last visit, time of intake or since the onset of the condition. The fourth question is about the pain level at it's worst, since the last visit, time of intake or since the onset of the condition. In order to assess the intensity of the pain, the answers for the four questions are treated as scores. The scores from factors 1,2,3, & 4 are averaged and multiplied by 10 to yield a score from $0 - 100$.

Reliability of the Tools Used

The Questionnaire used in the investigation was a standard type; Oswestry Low back pain Disability Questionnaire, which had been used for a lot of back pain studies, done in India and abroad. Fritz and Irrang[3], Davidson and Keating [4], Bayar et.al[5] have conducted studies with regard to the reliability

---

[3] Julie.M.Fritz, James.J.Irrang, A comparison of the modified Oswestry LBP disability questionnaire and the Quebec back pain disability scale, Physical Therapy, Vol.81 No.2 Feb.2001, pp 776-788

[4] Megan Davidson, Jennifer.L.Keating, A comparison of five Low back disability questionnaire; Reliability and responsiveness; Physical Therapy, Vol.82, No.1 Jan.2002, pp.8-24

and responsiveness of this questionnaire and discovered that the measurement obtained with modified Oswestry disability questionnaire was the most reliable and had sufficient width scale to reliably detect improvement/ worsening of the pain in subjects under study. Hence the reliability of the Questionnaire was ensured.

The Modified Schober's Test is a globally accepted test to assess the range of Spinal flexion and the same has been advised by Dr. Ronald Mcrae[6] and other eminent Orthopaedic experts like Lawrence.M.Tierney, Steepen.J.Mcphee, and Maxine.A.Papadakis [7]. Also studies done by R Williams, J Binkley and R.Bloch [8] and Viitanen.J.V. et al [9] and Moll and

---

[5] Bayar et.al, Reliability and Construct validity of the Oswestry Low Back Pain Disability Questionnaire, The Pain Clinic, Vol.15, No.1, 2003, pp.55-59

[6] Ronald McRae, Clinical Orthopeadic Examination, (Fifth Edition), Churchill Livingstone, Edinburgh, 2004, P.149

[7] Lawrence.M.Tierney, Steepen.J.Mcphee, Maxine.A.Papadakis, Current Medical Diagnosis & Treatment, Lange Medical Books/McGraw Hill, New York, 2004, P.789,

[8] R.Williams, J.Binkley, R.Bloch; Reliability of the modified Schober test for measuring lumbar flexion and extension, Physical Therapy, Vol. 73, No.1, January 1993, PP.33-44

[9] Viitanen.JV and Heikkila.S, Clinical Assessment of Spinal Mobility Measurements., Clinical Rheumatology, 2000, 19: 131-137

Wright [10] have proved the reliability of the modified Schober's test. Hence the test is found as reliable.

Quadruple Visual Analogue Scale also is used worldwide for rating the pain, which is an internationally accepted rating scale for back pain. Studies conducted by Von Korff & Deyo.R.A.[11], and Scrimshaw.SV & Maher.C [12], using this scale have proved it's reliability.

Tester's Competency & Reliability of Data

The Investigator, a college Lecturer in Physical Education who is very much interested in the academic field of Health Science, had gone through various books, journals/ periodicals and web sites in search of in-depth knowledge about the topic; "the influence of Yogic practices, Naturopathic and Physiotherapy treatment on low back pain patients".

The Yogic practices were given to the subjects by a trained Yoga practitioner and the Investigator has assisted the trainer in providing yogasanas

---

[10] Moll, J.M., & Wright.V., Normal range of spinal mobility: An objective clinical study. Annals of the Rheumatic Diseases, 1971, 30, 381-386.

[11] Von Korff.M., Deyo.R.A.,Cherkin.D., Back Pain in primary care; outcomes at 1 year, Spine:No.18, 1993,855-862

[12] Scrimshaw.SV, Maher.C, Responsiveness of Quadruple Visual Analogue Scale, Journal of.Manipulative and Physiological Therapeutics, 2001 Oct.24(8), 501-514

to the subjects. after she. herself underwent training of the various selected yogasanas in a reputed yoga center at Cochin for the purpose of this research. Similarly the Naturopathic treatment module has been designed by the Investigator with the guidance of the qualified Naturopaths of three Naturopathy centers at Cochin and the same has been provided to the subjects by the above Naturopathy centers. where the Investigator has assisted the Naturopaths. The Physiotherapy treatment modalities also has been chosen by the Investigator with the guidance of the qualified Physiotherapists of two major hospitals in Cochin City. The Investigator had assisted the Physiotherapists in providing various treatments and exercises to the subjects under study. Overall the Investigator joined hands with the Yoga Practictioners, Naturopaths and Physiotherapists in all the concerned activities with regard to the experiments, so as to get accurate results. Because of these factors, the Investigator is competent to conduct this study.

To establish the reliability of the data and tester's competency, a sample of 10 subjects were selected by the Investigator. The same tests were conducted on this sample by an Expert. The correlation coefficient was found out for the test conducted by the Investigator and the Expert. The correlation coefficient obtained indicated a value of 0.95, thereby establishing the competency of the tester to conduct the test and also proved the reliability of the data.

Subject Reliability

The Subjects were primarily self-referred and screened by a panel of Experts/ primary care physicians for inclusion/exclusion criteria.

Inclusion criteria for subjects, who were chosen for the study were as follows:

- mentally competent subjects aged between 30 & 60 years, normal on pre-study physical examination.

- Acute and chronic pain in the lower back.

- Radiating pain to the leg below the knee;

- Severity of symptoms 1 and above on the visual analogue scale from 0 (no pain) to 10 (worst possible pain);

- Duration of symptoms more than 10 weeks;

Subjects were excluded for the following reasons:

- Lower Back surgery had been performed in the previous 3 years;

- Epidural injection treatments had taken place in the past;

- Patient was pregnant;

- Indication for surgery was present at baseline (eg. progression of paresis or presence of cauda equina syndrome).

- had serious medical or psychiatric conditions, or had work schedules that were incompatible with the treatment schedule.

Instrument Reliability

All the instruments used in Physiotherapy treatment were quality instruments which were purchased from reputed companies by the Hospitals and the same were periodically caliberated The instruments had been used on two different occasions on the same sample subjects and the readings obtained on these two occasions showed a high correlation, thereby establishing instrument reliability.

Sampling and Recruitment:

Recruitment of the subjects (100 Nos.) for the study was facilitated by Life yoga center, Kochi, T.G.Chidhambaran Yoga Research Institute, Kochi, Cardinal Padiyara memorial Nature cure center, Kochi, Netaji Naturopathic research center, Kakkanad, Kochi, Sadhu Sevana Sabha Nature Cure Center, Moozhikkulam, Ernakulam, Physiotherapy Departments of Lissie Hospital and Lourdes Hospital Kochi. Interested patients were encouraged by the above centers to contact the Investigator directly, either by phone or e-mail and provide their name, phone number, and mailing address. Then an Information kit, which contained a sample consent form, a Backgrounder explaining the purpose of the study, a description of Yogic Practices/ Naturopathic Modalities/ Physiotherapy Techniques, was sent to each of these interested parties.

Following the mailing of the Information Kit, interested participants were contacted by telephone, and scheduled for a 1 hour initial consultation, in which any outstanding questions have been answered by the Investigator in the presence of the trained Yoga Practitioner/ Naturopath/ qualified Physiotherapist. A consent form has been signed by the subject and the intake interview and physical examination to evaluate the eligibility for the study, has been taken place. Eligible participants (20 each) were randomly assigned to either the Yoga group or Naturopathy group or Physiotherapy group or Combined group of Yoga & Naturopathy or the Control group.

3.6   EXPERIMENTAL TREATMENT DETAILS

Selected Yogic Practices (Noukasana, Leghu-Pavanamukthasana, Bhujangasana, Janusirasana, Ardh-Salabhasana, Merudandasana, Vakrasana and Vajramudra) were provided to the subjects for 1 hour daily and for seven days, in a week, in the case of Yoga group. Naturopathic treatment has been given to Naturopathy group, which included naturopathic diet (herbal drink, raw vegetable salad, fresh fruits and fruit juices, lemon juice, steamed vegetables, nuts, raw rice with sufficient bran) and baths like sun bath, hip bath, spinal bath and mud bath and massage as well as simple aerobic exercise like walking. Physiotherapy treatment (which consisted of Interferential current therapy (IFT), Short wave Diathermy, Ultra sound therapy, Lumbar Traction, Moist Hot packs, Transcutaneous electrical nerve stimulation (TENS), Infra red radiation, Massage and guidence on postural corrections) has been administered to the Physiotherapy group. Mckenzie Back extension exercises and Williams' Flexion exercises were also provided in the case of Physiotherapy group. Combined treatment of Yogic practices and Naturopathy have been provided to Yoga & Naturopathy group. The Control group has been kept as such and with out any kind of treatment. The various practices and treatment have been given for all the groups, for a specific duration of Twelve weeks. In the case of the Control group also, the observation period was twelve weeks.

3.6.1 DESCRIPTION OF THE TREATMENT ADMINISTERED TO YOGA GROUP

Iyengar has prescribed around fifty two yogic practices as curative asanas for low back pain.[13]

Out of these, the investigator selected eight asanas which were found most suitable for the subjects with mild/ moderate/ acute/ chronic low back ache, depends upon their age, general health condition, intensity of pain etc. In the case of some of the patients, all the eight asanas were not administered since one or two asanas were found little bit difficult for them to practice. In the case

---

[13] Iyengar.B.K.S., Light on Yoga, Harper Collins Publishers India, New Delhi, (thirty fourth edn.), 2006, PP.501-504

of others, selected asanas were provided in consideration of their pain intensity and other difficulties. However the subjects were administered with a minimum of six asanas. The Investigator herself had undergone yoga training in a reputed yoga center (Life Yoga Center, Cochin), for the purpose of this research and assisted the trained yoga practitioner of 'Life Yoga Center' in providing selected yogasanas to the subjects.

Preliminary precautions and Schedule of Yogic session

Time schedule :- 06.45 AM – 07.45 AM

Before starting to practice asana, the bladder was emptied and the bowels evacuated. Asanas come easier after taking bath. Taking a bath both before and after practicing asanas, refreshes the body and the mind. Asanas were done preferably on an empty stomach. If necessary, a cup of tea or boiled fresh milk was taken before the asanas. Asanas were practiced without discomfort and annoyance. Food has been taken half an hour after completing the asanas.

Asanas were done in clean airy place, free from insects and noise. It was done in a folded blanket laid on a leveled floor. No undue strain is left in the facial muscles, ears, eyes or in breathing during the practice. In the beginning keep the eyes open. The subject keeps the eyes closed only when he/she is perfect in a particular asana and then the subject is able to adjust the bodily movement and feel the correct stretching. During the practice, it is the body alone which is active while the brain remains passive, watchful and alert. In all the asanas the breathing was done through the nostrils only and not through the mouth.

During the practice period. the subjects took only "satwik foods" (preferably with sufficient vegetables and fruits). No alcoholic drinks was consumed during the practice period. The subjects were taking fresh nutritious food which was not so hot or so cold. The food which is kept in the refrigerator was avoided, even if it has been subjected to warming. Female subjects were advised to restrain from the practice during their menstural days.

For an acute phase of pain, yoga is not appropriate for 48 hours or until the acute period passes. If a yoga pose causesd any pain, tingling, or numbness, the practice of that particular asana was stopped immediately. The subjects were advised to move into the poses slowly and gently; used long holding times and practiced slow deep breathing in the poses. Any movements that increased the symptoms of the patients were avoided. The following yogic practices were given to the subjects for one hour daily, for a period of twelve weeks.

3.6.1.1 Naukasana

Technique

1. Lie down on the back. Keep the whole body loose and in a straight position. Palms can be on the floor. Keep the eyes gently closed with the

facial muscles relaxed and breathe deeply and slowly through the nostrils.

2. Exhale, recline the trunk back and simultaneously raise the legs from the floor, keeping the knees tight and toes pointed. The balance of the body rests on the buttocks and no part of the spine should be allowed to touch the floor.

3. At this stage the individual feels the grip on the muscles of the abdomen and the lower back.

4. Keep the legs at ankle of about 30° to 35° from the floor and the crown of the head in line with the toes.

5. Hold this pose for 20 to 30 seconds with normal breathing. A stay for one minute in this posture indicates strong abdominal muscles.

6. Do not hold the breath during this asana, though the tendency is always to do it with suspension of breath after inhalation.

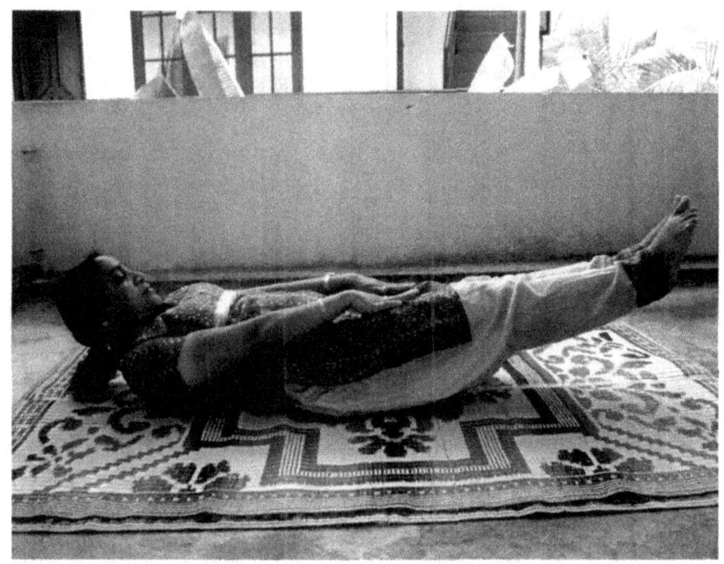

The Investigator demonstrating **NOUKASANA**

Therapeutic Effects

In the beginning, the back is too weak to bear the strain of the pose. When power to retain the pose comes, it indicates that the back is gaining strength. The asana helps to strengthen the lower back and thus reduces back pain.

3.6.1.2 Leghu Pavanamukthasana

Technique

1. Lie down on the floor with the face upward. Bend one of the knees and wrap the hands around the leg as shown in the posture.

2. Ensure that the hands are locked with the support of fingers.

3. Exhale slowly, raise the head forward till the forehead is nearer to the knee. The thigh should be pressed against the stomach.

4. Inhale and bring the forehead near the knees. Repeat the process for about 10 times.

5. Inhale deeply and gradually, then lower the head and relax.

6. This exercise is performed on each side, wherein each thigh presses against the stomach.

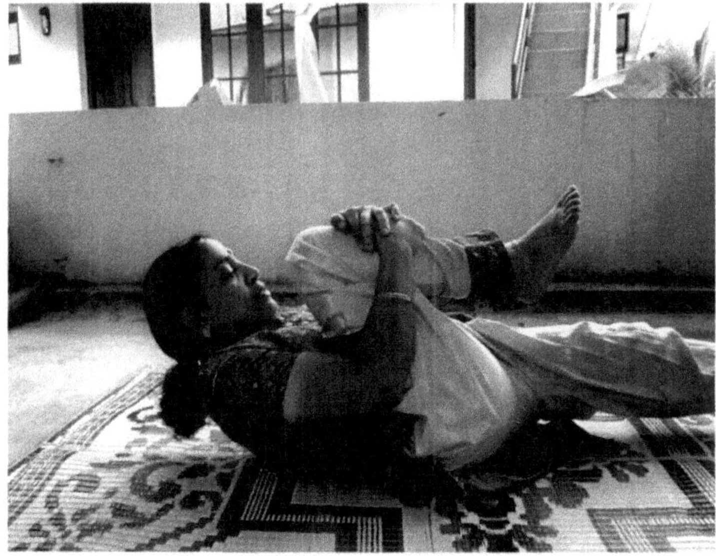

The Investigator demonstrating **LEKHU PAVANAMUKTHASANA**

Therapeutic Effects

This asana creates a better circulation of blood around the abdomen and the lower back. The dorsal region of the spine is very much exercised in this pose. Also the pose gives sufficient elasticity to the lower back which inturn minimizes the back ache.

3.6.1.3 Ardh Salabhasana

Technique

1. Lie on the abdomen with the chin touching the floor.

2. Push the chin a little more forward to bring the throat parallel to ground.

3. Then make fists of the hands and place them under the thighs with elbows close to each other. Keeping the hands beneath the body and chin pushed forward, inhale and raise the left leg up as high as possible.

4. Remember to keep the hips firm on the floor and the knees straight.

5. Now bring down the leg gently and repeat the process with the other leg. The individual can keep on holding up each leg for up to 15 seconds.

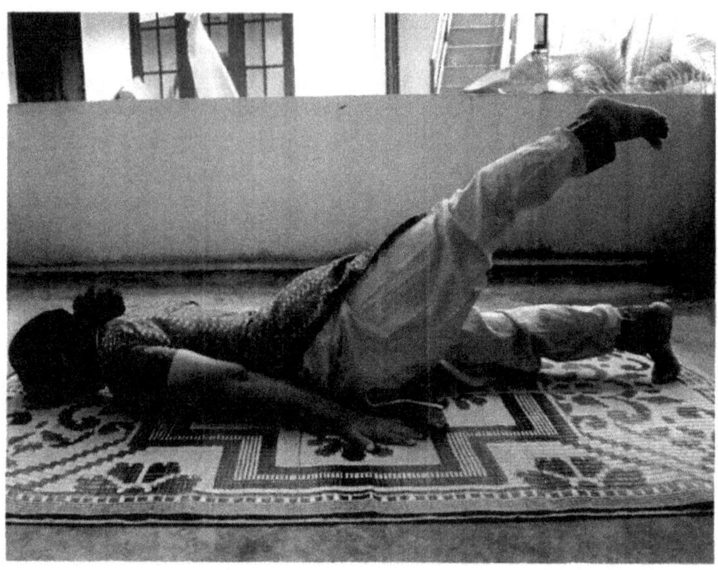

The Investigator demonstrating **ARDH SALABHASANA**

Therapeutic Effects

Since the spine is stretched back, it becomes elastic and the pose relieves pain in the sacral and lumbar regions.

3.6.1.4 Bhujangasana

Technique

1. Lie on the floor, face downwards. Extend the legs, keeping the feet together. Keep the knees tight and the toes pointing.

2. Rest the palms by the side of the pelvic region.

3. Inhale and press the palms firmly on the floor and pull the trunk up. Take two breaths.

4. Inhale, lift the body up from the trunk until the pubis is in contact with the floor. Stay in this position with the weight of the legs and palms.

5. Contract the annus and the buttocks, tighten the thighs.

6. Maintain the pose for about 20 seconds, breath normally.

7. Exhale, bent the elbows and rest the trunk on the floor. Repeat the pose two or three times and then relax.

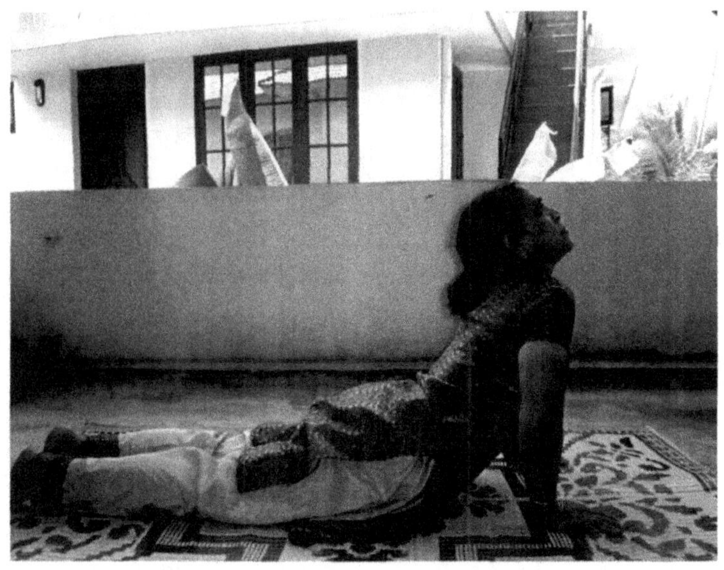

The Investigator demonstrating **BHUJANGASANA**

Therapeutic Effects

The posture is a panacea for an injured spine and in case of slight displacement of the spinal discs, the practice of this pose replaces the discs in their original position. The spine region is toned and thereby the pain is reduced.

3.6.1.5 Merudandasana

Technique

1. Lie on the back. Legs should touch each other and palms should rest on the ground on each side of the body.

2. Take a deep breath and raise the legs to more than 2 feet from the ground. The knees should be straight.

3. Hold the breath for five seconds. Slowly exhale and bring the legs to the ground.

4. Repeat the asanas for ten times.

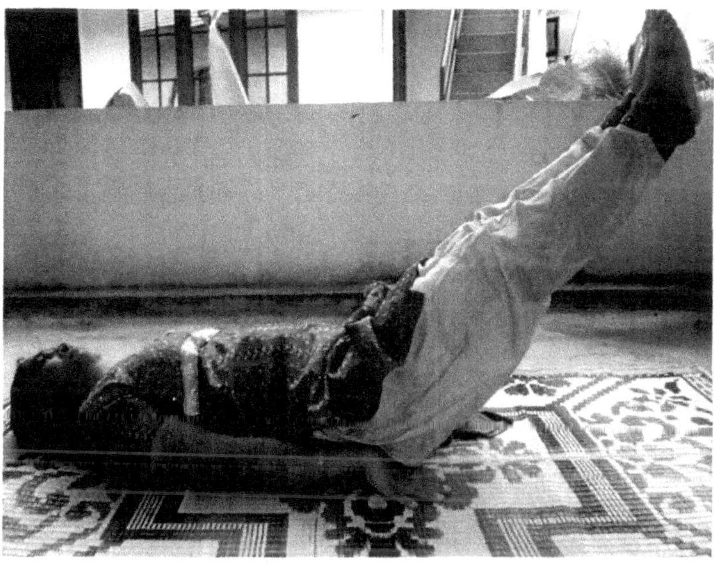

The Investigator demonstrating **MERUDANDASANA**

Therapeutic Effects

This strengthens the vertebrae and stop the accumulation of fat in the lower stomach region. This asana keeps the dorsal portion of the spine supple and healthy. It tones the lower back by ensuring with the supply of healthy blood and thereby reduces back ache.

3.6.1.6 Vakrasana

Technique

1. Sit erect, stretching the legs in front together. Hands by the side, palm resting on the ground, fingers together pointing forward.

2. Slowly fold right leg at the knee and place the sole on the ground near the knee of the left leg. The knee of the right leg should make 90° angle straight towards sky.

3. Taking the right hand towards back, place the palm on the ground at the distance of 9" straight from spine. Fingers together pointing backward. Then place the left hand towards the other side of the right knee.

4. Now twist the head and back towards backside and try to look at the backside.

5. While returning to the original position first bring the head to the orginal position.

6. Now take the left hand to its original position and then bring the right hand from the back and place it by the side of the body.

7. Now slowly stretch out the folded leg and sit erect as in the first position.

8. In the same way, practice it from the other leg. This makes one round of Vakrasana.

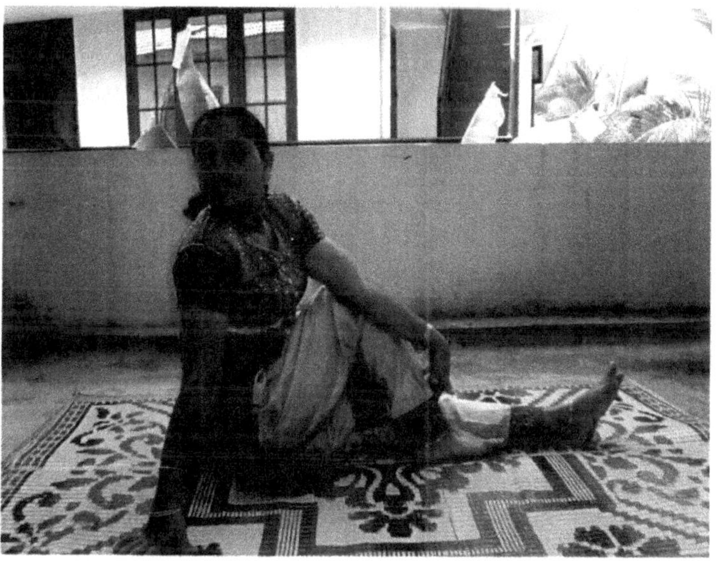

The Investigator demonstrating **VAKRASANA**

Therapeutic Effects

In this posture the spine is stretched. This asana brings back elasticity to the spine and tones the abdominal organs and thereby minimizes low back pain.

3.6.1.7 Janusirasana

Technique

1 Get into the sitting position of Sukhasana.

2 Stretch out the legs in front of the body. Spread the legs while keeping the heels apart. The heels should be about 15 inches away from each other.

3 Slide the left foot back while bending the left knee outwards. Rest the left knee on the floor.

4 Inhale and raise the arms above the head. Face the palms of the hands outwards.

5 Release all the air out of the body by exhaling completely. Stiffen the knees and inhaling deeply.

6 Exhale again and draw in the abdomen. Bend forwards from the waist with the upper portion of the body touching the right thigh. Extend forward and grip the left foot with both hands.

7 Take a deep breath and release it. On the exhale, press the right knee into the floor and bend the elbows out to push the upper body further down.

8 Rest the forehead on your right knee.

9　Gradually release the elbows and lay them on the floor. Make sure that the entire right leg is touching the floor.

10　Maintain this position while breathing normally. To come out of it, slowly reverse the above steps. Then repeat them with the left leg being stretched outwards.

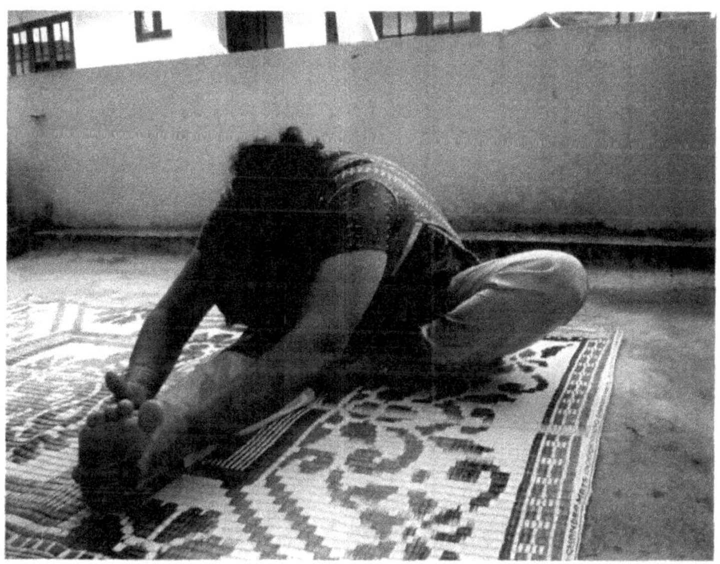

The Investigator demonstrating **JANUSIRASANA**

Therapeutic Effects

The pose stimulates the blood circulation to the spine and relieves low back ache. This is a very invigorating pose.

3.6.1.8 Vajramudra

Technique

1 Sit on the floor and bend the legs at the knees. Place the heels at the side of the anus in such a way that the thighs rests on the legs and the buttocks rest on the heels.

2 Support the whole body on the knees and the ankles. Slowly and cautiously bend the trunk forward.

3 Take the arms to the back. Hold the right forearm with the left hand and the left forearm with the right hand.

4 Inhale. Slowly exhale and stretch the neck downwards, so that the nose touches the ground. Do this for a time limit of ten seconds.

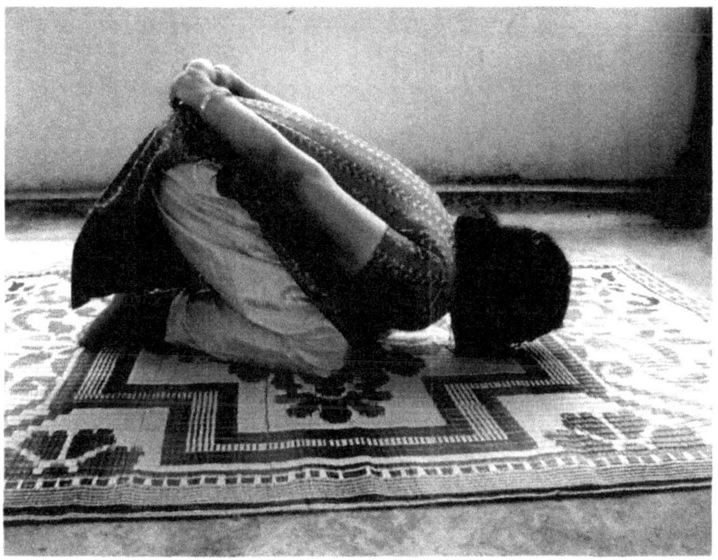

The Investigator demonstrating **VAJRAMUDRA**

Therapeutic Effects

This asana tones the lower back since the back muscle are exercised and thereby the lower back feel soothed. It also ensure with the supply of healthy blood to the lower back and thus reduces back ache.

3.6.2 DESCRIPTION OF THE TREATMENT ADMINISTERED TO NATUROPATHY GROUP

The investigator referred a number of authentic books and journals/periodicals on naturopathy for getting idea about the right kind of naturopathic food suitable for low back pain patients. The investigator consulted practicing naturopaths of three naturopathy centers at Ernakulam also, for getting an overall idea about the naturopathic diet. Then the investigator developed a unique Naturopathic Treatment module which comprised absolute naturopathic diet, herbal drink, various baths, massage, meditation, pranayama, prayer and exercise, which have curative effect on low back pain patients and the same is given below.

3.6.2.1 NATUROPATHIC TREATMENT MODULE (IN DETAIL)

Time	Details of Diet & other Programmes
06 00 AM	Herbal Drink – 180 ml
06 10 AM	Prayer, Meditation & Pranayama (30 minutes)
07 00 AM	HIP BATH – 15 minutes
07 30 AM	**BREAK FAST** (Vegetable soup *, Germinated pulses (Bengai gram) & Fresh Fruits **) – (Soup - 180 ml, Pulses - 100 gm, Fruits - 300 gm)
08 15 AM	SUN BATH – 15 minutes

09 00 AM	Herbal Drink – 180 ml
09 10 AM	SPINAL BATH - 20 minutes
11.00 AM	Lemon juice – 180 ml
11.15 AM	Massage (Naturopathic massage of lower back)
00 00 PM	**LUNCH :-** 2 whole wheat chappathi plus steamed vegetables (vegetables include carrot, cabbage, tomato, raddish & beet root – 40 gms each)
	REST
02 00 PM	Fresh Fruit Juice – 200 ml (Orange / Apple/ Pine apple)
02 05 PM	MUD BATH – 1 hour
03 05 PM	Herbal Drink – 180 ml
03 10 PM	HIP BATH - 15 minutes
03 45 PM	Fresh Fruits (Apple & Pappaya – 200 gm)
04 00 PM	SUN BATH – 15 minutes
05 00 PM	Nuts (Badam [Almond] & Walnut) – 40 gms/ Dates (dried) – 50 gms (dates & nuts, alternate days).
05 30 PM	HIP BATH – 15 minutes
06 00 PM	Herbal Drink – 180 ml
06 15 PM	Walking (as an aerobic exercise) – 30 minutes ***
08 00 PM	**DINNER ******
09 00 PM	Sleep

* Beans, Cabbage, Cauliflower and Spinach to form the soup.

** Fruits for break fast consists of orange, pineapple and grape fruit.

*** Weight bearing exercises such as walking, help to strengthen the bones. The weight bearing load increases the calcium deposits in the bones, thus increases the bone density and reduce the risk for Osteoporosis.

**** Boiled raw Rice having sufficient bran, Raw Vegetable Salad with Carrot, Tomato & Cucumber) and boiled Vegetables (Beans, lettuce, cauliflower and spinach)

Herbal Drink (Preparation)

Coriander	-	100 gm
Cumin	-	20 gm
Fenugreek	-	20 gm
Ginger (dried) powder	-	10 gm
Cardamom	-	5 gm

Coriander, Cumin and Fenugreek have to be fried and then powdered. To this add dried Ginger powder and Cardamom powder. This will form a mixture and take 3 gm. out of this and add to a glass of water (180 ml). Then boil it with 15 gms of palm jaggery for sweetness.

3.6.2.2 Effects of Herbal Drink

Coriander is diuretic in nature (helps to remove the excess fluid present in the body by way of increasing the urine production), and has analgesic & anti-inflammatory properties. The Fenugreek has anti arthritic property, which heals disorders like spondylosis. Cumin is also diuretic in nature and it decreases the excess fluid in the body, especially in the lungs, ankles and legs. Ginger is anti inflammatory & analgesic and hence reduces pain.

Details of the Naturopathic Diet, it's Caloric value, Calcium & Vitamin C contents (Refer Appendix – ii)

Table for <u>Male subjects</u> (K. Calories required - 2400/ day)

Calcium requirement: 1000 - 1100 mg/day

Diet	K.Calories	Calcium (mg)	Vitamin C (mg)
Herbal Drink – 180 ml x 4 glasses	269	80	16
BREAK FAST (Vegetable soup, * Germinated pulses (Bengal gram) & Fresh Fruits **) – (Soup 180 ml, Pulses - 120 gm, Fruits - 300 gm)	533	324	143
Lemon juice (180 ml)	57	70	39
Fresh Fruit Juice – 200 ml	29	15	44

(Grapes/Orange/Pine apple) – Average (Alternate days)			
LUNCH ***	517	330	94
Nuts & Dates – dried (Nuts include 20 gm each of Almond & Walnut and 50 gm of Dates)	408	97	0
Dinner ****	588	158	28
	2401	**1074**	**364**

* Beans, Cabbage, Cauliflower and Spinach (25 gm each) and the rest water, to form the soup.

** Fruits for break fast include Apple & Pappaya (150 gm each)

*** Lunch consists of 2 ½ whole wheat chappathi (125 gm) & steamed vegetables (40 gm each of carrot, tomato, & radish, 60 gm each of beet root & cabbage)

**** Dinner consists of Raw Rice (150 gm), raw salad (50 gm each of tomato & cucumber) and half cooked carrot, cabbage, beans, cauliflower & beet root (25 gm each)

Details of the Naturopathic Diet, it's Caloric value, Calcium &

Vitamin C contents (Refer Appendix – ii)

Table for <u>Female subjects</u> (K. Calories required - 2100/ day)

Calcium requirement: 1000 - 1100 mg/day

Diet	K.Calories	Calcium mg	Vitamin C mg
Herbal Drink – 180 ml x 4 glasses	268	80	16
BREAK FAST (Vegetable soup, * Germinated pulses (Bengal gram) & Fresh Fruits **) – (Soup - 180 ml, Pulses - 120 gm, Fruits - 300 gm)	531	324	143
Lemon juice (180 ml)	57	70	39
Fresh Fruit Juice – 200 ml (Grapes/Orange/Pine apple) – Average	29	15	44
LUNCH ***	430	320	94
Nuts & Dates – dried (Nuts include 20 gm each of Almond & Walnut and 50 gm of Dates)	408	97	0
Dinner ****	413	153	28
	2136	1059	364

* Beans, Cabbage, Cauliflower and Spinach (25 gm each) and the rest water, to form the soup.

** Fruits for break fast consists of Apple & Pappaya (150 gm each)

*** Lunch consists of 2 whole wheat chappathi (100 gm) & steamed vegetables (40 gm each of carrot, tomato, & radish, 60 gm each of beet root & cabbage)

**** Dinner consists of Raw Rice (100 gm), raw salad (50 gm each of tomato & cucumber) and half cooked carrot, cabbage, beans, cauliflower & beet root (25 gm each)

3.6.2.3 Effects of Fruits and Vegetables

On naturopathic diet, the patients with low back pain enjoy a beneficial increase in the vitamin C intake. Recent research work has pointed out a possible protective role of vitamin C. An important component of all connective tissues is a substance known as hyaluronic acid, which strengthens the synovial membranes of the joints and checks the spread of infectious agents and inflammatory substances such as histamine. When hyaluronic acid is in short supply, there is an increased risk of arthritis or bleeding into the joints. Painful arthritic swelling of the joints can also result from an excessive activity of hyaluronidase, the naturally occuring substance which is responsible for the breakdown of the hyaluronic acid in the body. This may occur as a direct result of vitamin C deficiency.

An anti-backache diet is one which contains lot of vitamin C. This can be achieved by eating fresh citrous fruits (Orange, Grapes, Pineapple), which contains lot of vitamin C everyday, together with plenty of salads and lightly cooked green vegetables. A diet designed for low back pain patients also contain an adequate allowance of calcium and vitamin D, the nutrients which are essential for the formation of strong healthy bones. Calcium, magnesium and sodium are the essential minerals, human beings require for bone building. The naturopathic diet prescribed above, provide these minerals sufficiently.

Bone and Cartilage strengthening vitamins such as Vitamin C & Vitamin D are obtained from naturopathic diet. Minerals such as calcium, magnesium and manganese which are essential for bone strengthening are also obtained from naturopathic way of food habits. Bromelain, the enzyme found in pineapple helps to reduce inflammation and pain from trauma, sports injuries and arthritis.

Lemon Juice

It contains substantial quantity of Vitamin C. It is sour in taste but it's reaction in the human body is alkaline and as such it is valuable in rheumatic afflictions. The lemon juice prevents the deposit of uric acid in the tissues. Vitamin C is necessary for the development of healthy bone metrix. Vitamin D, Calcium, Phosphorus and the essential trace minerals are required for healthy bones. Vitamin C has proved helpful in relieving back pain and averting spinal disc operations.

3.6.2.4 Spinal Bath (Hot)

The Spinal bath is an important form of hydrotherapic treatment. This is carried out in a tub, having around four feet length and two feet width. Hot water (103 – 105° FH) is filled in the tub upto four inches height. Then the individual lie in the tub, placing both the legs and head out side the tub, for about 20 minutes. Throughout the bath, the temperature of the water is maintained at 103-105° F.

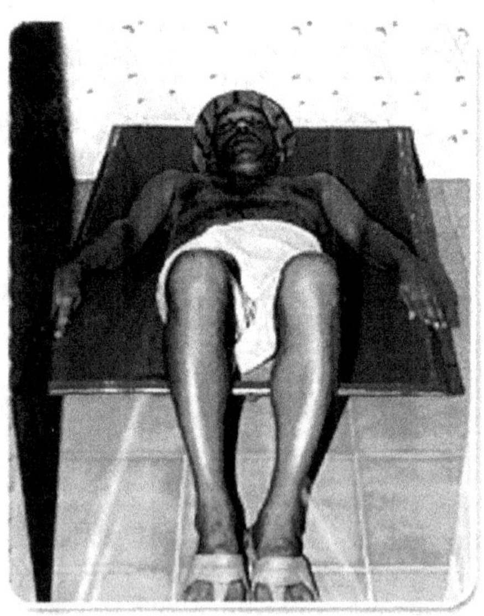

Effects

Hot Bath soothe the cutanious nerves and nerves of internal organs in reflex relation with the skin areas to which the heat is applied. Hot Bath relaxes tissues including the cappillaries of the skin which draws blood from the deeper tissues. Hot Bath stimulates the nerves and also relieves pain including at the lower back. The bath provides a soothing effect to the spinal column. The hot spinal bath relieves vertebral pain due to spondylitis and muscular pain in the lower back. It also relieves sciatic pain. As a result of the bath, the blood circulation increases to the lower back which in turn relieves the pain.

3.6.2.5 Hip Bath (Hot)

Hip bath is carried out in a tub, having two feet diameter. Water is filled in the tub up to six inches in height, Then the individual may sit in the tub in a slanding position, adjuscent to the wall, for about 15 minutes. Thin persons should take it for only 15 minutes and the stout persons can continue for 20 minutes. The water temperature is maintained at 40 – 45°C. The bath starts at 40°C and then the temperature is gradually increased to 45°C. Then throughout the bath, the temperature of the water is maintained at 45°C. Before entering the tub, the patient drinks one glass of cold water. A cold compress should be placed on the head. The individual take a rough towel and rubs the abdomen gently from the right to the left. A cold shower bath is taken immediately after the hot hip bath. Care is taken to prevent the patient from catching a chill after the bath. In the beginning, Hip bath is taken only for five to eight minutes. The time is increased gradually day by day.

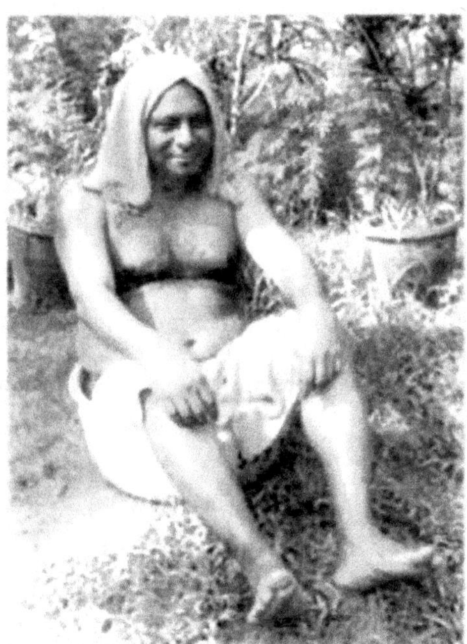

Effects

The Hip Bath (hot) helps to relieve muscular spasm and lower back pain due to Sciatica. The warmth of water relieves pain and muscle spasm and promote relaxation. As in the case of spinal bath, here also the blood circulation increases to the lower back as a result of the bath, which in turn relieves the pain. Hot Bath stimulates the nerves and also relieves pain at the lower back.

3.6.2.6 Sun Bath

Sun Bath is done when the sun has risen some what high in the sky and it's heat is mild, ie within three hours after sun rise. The patient lies down on a bed sheet spread on the ground, covered with a thin dry cloth on the body, till he gets warmed and then he uses a wet cloth by replacing the dry cloth. If the face also be in the sun, it is covered with a folded wet cloth. The patient begins with 3 to 4 minutes of this bath and gradually increases it up to 15 minutes. After this, the skin surface is wrapped clean with a nearly dry wet cloth.

Effects

The sun bath is much beneficial to osteoporotic patients. Vitamin D is necessary for maintaining a normal blood concentration of calcium. It also enhances the absorption of calcium from the intestines. Vitamin D is manufactured in the body from a precursor molecule that is produced when the skin is exposed to direct sunlight. It is a natural source of Vitamin D, which is inevitable for the growth and stregthening of the bones. Vitamin D helps calcium and Phosphorous to build bones. Vitamin D is formed in the skin, by the activity of the ultra violet rays in the sun light.

3.6.2.7 Mud Bath (Mud Pack)

In Mud bath, clay taken from about four inches below the surface of the earth is used. It is ensured that the clay does not contain any impurities like compost or pebbles. Mix it with cold water so as to get a consistancy like soft dough. It should stick and not be thin enough to slide down, when used in the pack. The mud is   thickly applied on the body part (lower back) which requires treatment. The patient is then wrapped in towel or sheet and remains in the mud envolope for one hour. The mud is then washed off with a spray and the skin is rapidly dried. Then bath is taken at 100°F to 104°F.

Effects

The cold moisture in the mud packs relaxes the pores of the skin, draws blood into the surface, relieves inner congestion and pain and promotes heat radiation and thus eliminate morbid matter from the body of the patient.

3.6.2.8 Naturopathic Massage

The patient is made to lie down with the arms at the sides. The masseur effleurages the lower back using both hands on each sides of the spine. Stroking is done from the sacrum upwards. Friction follows with each hand at the sides of the spine going down slowly. Kneading by muscle picking is done with squeezing. Then the masseur carries out alternate rapid pushing and pulling movements of the hands sliding down the spine. Circular kneading also is done.

The treatment ends by slapping, hacking and cupping at each side of the spine.

In Naturopathic massage, Mustard oil is used to minimise low back pain.

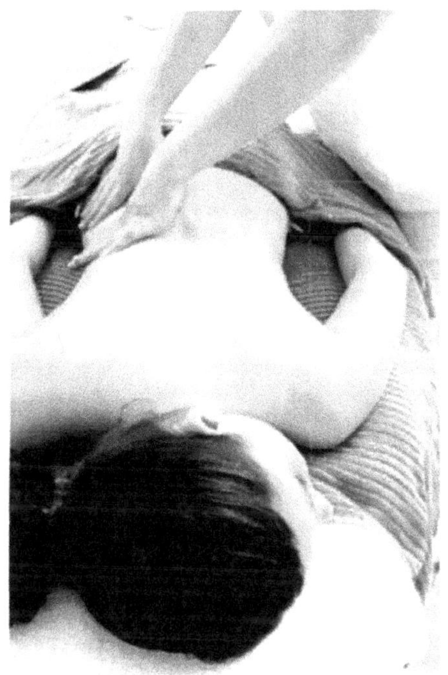

Effects

Gentle stroking and light kneading of the lower back is pain relieving and soothing. Percussion and vibration result into stimulating experience.

Vibration of the end of the spine benefits the sacral nerves. It is beneficial in toning the muscles and the tendons of the joints. It reduces the pain, redness and swelling which are the cardinal signs of the inflammation. In massage the muscles get regenerated and are then capable of holding half of the blood supply. Massage thus provides additional nourishment to feed the muscular tissues, helping them to grow strong. Tapping, striking and vibrating help the muscles to develop it's contractile power.

3.6.2.9 Low impact Aerobic Exercise

Engaging in a low-impact exercise program (like walking) aids to maintain everyday functionality. Back pain patients are engaged in walking as it is easy on the joints and gentle on the back.

Effects

Exercise improves the supply of nutrients to spinal discs, and thereby delaying the process of deterioration that comes with age.

Other Guidelines in Naturopathic Treatment

While taking rest or while sleeping, the patient has been instructed to lie straight and as chest upwards, on wooden coat, without bed and pillows. The patient was also instructed to take care to be in a slanding position, while raising from the coat, by applying pressure on his/her hands. The patients slept on a firm mattress on their sides with knees bend at right angles to the torso.

Soft cushioned seats were avoided. The patient took care, never to bend from the waist down to lift any object, but instead squat close to the object, bending the knees, but keeping the back straight, and then stand up slowly.

In the case of combined treatment of Yogic practices and Naturopathy, the timings of yogic practices and naturopathic treatment have been adjusted appropriately, in the morning so as to accommodate the procedures of both the treatments in the most convenient way.

3.6.3 DESCRIPTION OF THE TREATMENT ADMINISTERED TO PHYSIOTHERAPY GROUP

The Physiotherapy treatment given to each patient in the group, differs in accordance with the symptoms, intensity of the pain, age etc. The brief schedule of the treatment administered to twenty subjects is given below.

Patient No.	Description of the Treatment given
1	Lumbar Traction – 20 minutes at a time (60 days) – Intermittently, by a gap of 3 days. Initially traction for 6 days, then a gap of 3 days, after that again traction for 6 days; then a gap of 3 days; like that 10 sessions. Interferential current Therapy (IFT) - 15 minutes. (20 days) Massage – 30 minutes (30 days). After one week started Mckenzie's Extension Exercises and afterwards Williams Flexion Exercises. Administered every exercises within the pain limit.

2	Lumbar Traction – 20 minutes at a time (48 days) – Intermittently, by a gap of 3 days. Initially traction for 6 days, then a gap of 3 days, after that again traction for 6 days; then a gap of 3 days; like that 8 sessions. Short Wave Diathermy (SWD) - 20 minutes. (15 days) Massage – 45 minutes (30 days) After one week, started Mckenzie's Extension Exercises and afterwards Williams Flexion Exercises. Administered every exercises within the pain limit.
3	Moist Hot Packs – 30 minutes. (20 days) Interferential current Therapy (IFT) - 15 minutes.(15 days) Ultra Sound Therapy – 10 minutes. (10 days) Massage – 30 minutes (20 days) After five days, started Mckenzie's Extension Exercises and afterwards Williams Flexion Exercises. Administered every exercises within the pain limit. Use Lumbar corset during long driving.
4	Lumbar Traction – 20 minutes at a time (60 days) – Intermittently, by a gap of 3 days. Initially traction for 6 days, then a gap of 3 days, after that again traction for 6 days; then a gap of 3 days; like that 10 sessions.

	Interferential current Therapy (IFT) - 15 minutes.(20 days) Massage – 30 minutes (30 days) After one week started Mckenzie's Extension Exercises and afterwards Williams Flexion Exercises. Administered every exercises within the pain limit. Avoid long journey, Two wheeler driving and weight lifting
5	Transcutaneous Electrical Nerve Stimulation (TENS) - 15 minutes. (21 days) Massage – 45 minutes. (20 days) Moist Hot Packs – 30 minutes.(15 days) After one week started Mckenzie's Extension Exercises and afterwards Williams Flexion Exercises. Administered every exercises within the pain limit.
6	Lumbar Traction – 20 minutes at a time (42 days) – Intermittently, by a gap of 3 days. Initially traction for 6 days, then a gap of 3 days, after that again traction for 6 days; then a gap of 3 days; like that 7 sessions. Infra Red radiation - 15 minutes.(3 weeks) Transcutaneous Electrical Nerve Stimulation(TENS) -15 minutes (20 days) Massage – 30 minutes (30 days)

		After 10 days started Mckenzie's Extension Exercises and afterwards Williams Flexion Exercises. Administered every exercises within the pain limit. Used Lumbar corset during prolonged standing.
	7	Infra red Radiation – 20 minutes (15 days) Massage – 45 minutes.(30 days) Moist Hot Packs – 30 minutes (20 days) After ten days, started Mckenzie's Extension Exercises and afterwards Williams Flexion Exercises. Administered every exercises within the pain limit.
	8	Interferential current Therapy (IFT) - 15 minutes. (20 days) Massage – 45 minutes (25 days) After ten days, started Mckenzie's Extension Exercises and afterwards Williams Flexion Exercises. Administered every exercises within the pain limit.

9	Short Wave Diathermy – 25 minutes (20 days) Ultra Sound Therapy – 10 minutes (15 days) Massage – 30 minutes (30 days) After one week started Mckenzie's Extension Exercises and afterwards Williams Flexion Exercises. Administered every exercises within the pain limit. Used Lumbar corset during driving
10	TENS - 15 minutes (20 days) Infra red Radiation – 20 minutes (15 days) After 5 days, started Mckenzie's Extension Exercises and afterwards Williams Flexion Exercises. Administered every exercises within the pain limit.
11	Interferential current Therapy (IFT) - 15 minutes. (20 days) Massage – 45 minutes (25 days) Moist Hot Packs – 30 minutes (20 days) After one week started Mckenzie's Extension Exercises and afterwards Williams Flexion Exercises. Administered every exercises within the pain limit. Used Lumbar corset during travelling and Driving

12	Lumbar Traction – 20 minutes at a time (36 days) – Intermittently, by a gap of 3 days. Initially traction for 6 days, then a gap of 3 days, after that again traction for 6 days; then a gap of 3 days; like that 6 sessions. Short Wave Diathermy – 20 minutes (14 days) Interferential current Therapy (IFT) - 15 minutes.(20 days) Massage – 30 minutes (20 days) After ten days started Mckenzie's Extension Exercises and afterwards Williams Flexion Exercises. Administered every exercises within the pain limit.
13	Infra red radiation – 15 minutes (15 days) Interferential current Therapy (IFT) - 15 minutes (14 days). Moist Hot Packs – 30 minutes (15 days) Massage – 40 minutes (30 days) After five days, started Mckenzie's Extension Exercises and afterwards Williams Flexion Exercises. Administered every exercises within the pain limit.
14	Massage – 40 minutes (20 days) TENS - 15 minutes. (20 days) Ultra sound Therapy – 8 minutes (15 days) After one week started Mckenzie's Extension Exercises and

		afterwards Williams Flexion Exercises. Administered every exercises within the pain limit. Used lumbar corset while travelling and during prolonged standing
15		Lumbar Traction – 20 minutes at a time (60 days) – Intermittently, by a gap of 3 days. Initially traction for 6 days, then a gap of 3 days, after that again traction for 6 days; then a gap of 3 days; like that 10 sessions. Infra red Radiation - 15 minutes (14 days) Massage – 30 minutes (25 days) After ten days, started Mckenzie's Extension Exercises and afterwards Williams Flexion Exercises. Administered every exercises within the pain limit.
16		Interferential current Therapy (IFT) - 15 minutes (14 days) Short wave Diathermy – 30 minutes (12 days) Massage – 45 minutes (20 days) After five days, started Mckenzie's Extension Exercises and afterwards Williams Flexion Exercises. Administered every exercises within the pain limit.
17		Interferential current Therapy (IFT) - 15 minutes (15 days) TENS – 15 minutes (12 days) Moist Hot Packs – 30 minutes (20 days)

	Massage – 30 minutes (30 days) After one week started Mckenzie's Extension Exercises and afterwards Williams Flexion Exercises. Administered every exercises within the pain limit.
18	Infra red Radiation – 20 minutes (10 days) Interferential current Therapy (IFT) - 15 minutes (10 days) Massage – 30 minutes (30 days) After five days, started Mckenzie's Extension Exercises and afterwards Williams Flexion Exercises. Administered every exercises within the pain limit. Used Lumbar corset during Driving.
19	Short Wave Diathermy – 25 minutes (12 days) Ultra sound Therapy – 7 minutes (15 days) Interferential current Therapy (IFT) - 15 minutes (14 days) Moist Hot Packs – 30 minutes (20 days) Massage – 30 minutes (40 days) After one week started Mckenzie's Extension Exercises and afterwards Williams Flexion Exercises. Administered every exercises within the pain limit.
20	TENS – 15 minutes (14 days) Infra red Radiation - 6 minutes (14 days)

<table>
<tr><td></td><td>

Massage – 30 minutes (30 days)

After 5 days, started Mckenzie's Extension Exercises and afterwards Williams Flexion Exercises. Administered every exercises within the pain limit.

Used lumbar corset while travelling and during prolonged standing

</td></tr>
</table>

General guidelines given to the Subjects, participated in the Physiotherapy Treatment

Care is taken, to have good posture always.

Use lumbar corset during long distance driving and during continous standing.

Avoid the use of belt during sleeping and while taking Food

Take sufficient rest during long journey. If the patient gets pain during long journey driving, change the sitting position and take rest for 10 minutes and relax and then continue driving.

Avoid over travelling , 2 wheeler journey and weight lifting.

Avoid heels and prolonged standing.

DETAILS OF VARIOUS PHYSIOTHERAPY TECHNIQUES APPLIED

3.6.3.1 Interferential therapy (IFT):

Interferential current therapy is a unique way of effectively delivering therapeutic frequencies to tissues. Interferential stimulators use a fixed carrier frequency of 4,000 Hz per sec. and also a second adjustable frequency of 4,001-4,400 Hz per second. When the fixed and adjustable frequencies combine (heterodyne), they produce the desired signal frequency (Interference frequency).Interferential stimulation is concentrated at the point of intersection between the electrodes. The Interferential stimulation is given for 15 minutes.

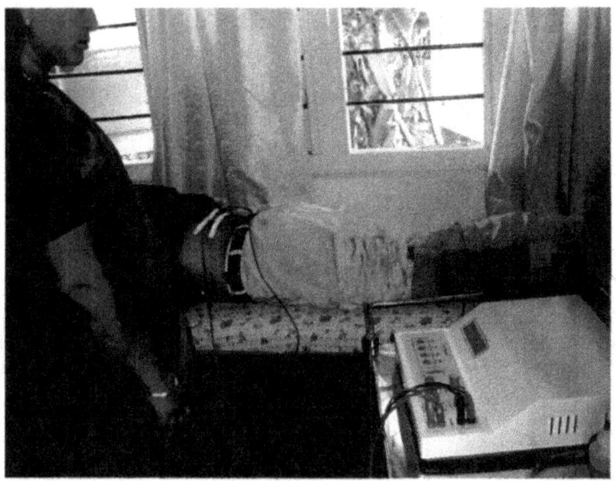

The Investigator Provides IFT treatment to the subject

Effects

In Interferential current therapy, current perfuses to greater depths and over a larger volume of tissues than other forms of electrical therapy. When current is applied to the skin, capacitive skin resistance decreases as pulse frequency increases. Interferential current crosses the skin with greater ease and with less stimulation of cutaneous nociceptors allowing greater patient comfort during electrical stimulation. In addition, because medium-frequency (Interferential) current is tolerated better by the skin, the dosage can be increased, thus improving the ability of the interferential current to permeate tissues and allowing easier access to deep structures. Interferential stimulation allows a deeper penetration of the tissue with more comfort (compliance) and increased circulation. The Interference frequencies interfere with the transmission of pain at the spinal cord level and the patient feels reduction in pain.

3.6.3.2 Computerized Lumbar Traction

Spinal Decompression therapy by way of computerized traction is designed to help patients who suffer from disc problems including bulging, herniated, or degenerated discs in the neck and low back. The Patient lies on the Decompression Table with comfortable pads behind their waist depending on their treatment. The computerized process involves a series of gentle stretches that separate the vertebrae causing a negative pressure in the disc. Because of this negative pressure, disc material which has protruded or herniated is pulled back within the normal confines of the disc and permit healing to occur.

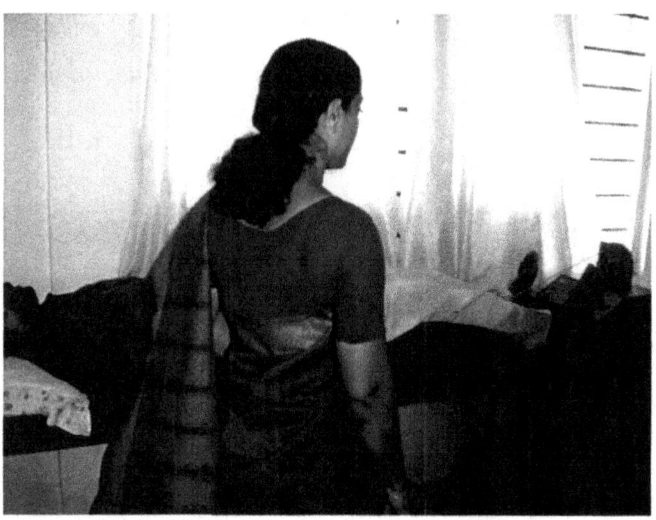

The Investigator Provides Lumbar Traction to the subject

Although these changes are almost imperceptible after each treatment, over time, the results are truly remarkable. The treatment plan is customized for each patient depending on his or her condition.

Decompression therapy adds progressively more tension until it arrives in the "treatment zone" where it gently pumps the disc. The computer connected with the instrument is the key. It controls the variations in the traction pull allowing for spinal decompression and eliminating muscle guarding that is typical in conventional traction devices. Traction might feel good to a patient who doesn't have a lot of pain or muscle tightness to begin with. The mechine utilizes a special table that "expands" and "contracts" as the spine is being decompressed. The result is a fluid motion that allows for high patient comfort and utilizes less force to produce the results.

Effects

The gentle pumping action utilized by the Decompression Table helps nutrient-rich fluids flow to the inside of the disc. This allows for additional healing to occur in the areas of disc degeneration. The pumping action involved in computerized traction promote a process called imbibition which pulls nutrients into the disc to maximize the health of this living, vital area of the spine.

3.6.3.3 SHORTWAVE DIATHERMY

This deep heat modality is the therapeutic application of high radio-frequency electrical currents. The radiofrequency electromagnetic field usually is at a frequency of 27.12 MHz (l=11.06 m). A transverse technique is applied to treat a larger anatomic area with the primary concentration at the mid point between electrodes.

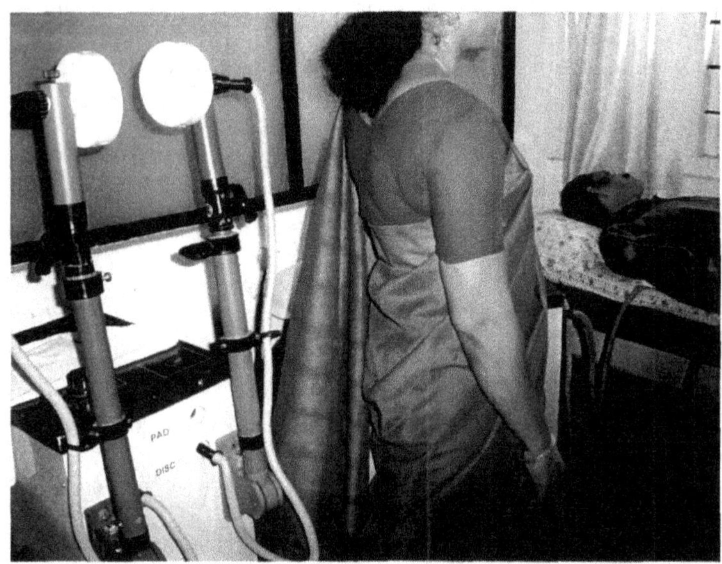

The Investigator Provides Short Wave Diathermy to the subject

Proper application and tuning are given in this process. The patient's electrical impedance becomes part of the impedance of the patient's own circuit. The patient's circuit is set to resonance, so the patient's circuit frequency is equal to that of the machine. The patient feels only a comfortable heat. The tissue temperature is elevated to a range of 40-45°C for therapeutic benefit. Continuous supervision and observation of the patient is done. The treatment time is usually 20-30 minutes. At clinically relevant energies, shortwave diathermy increases subcutaneous fat temperature 15°C and muscle 4-6°C at a depth of 4-5 cm. Application of this modality is restricted to patients on either wooden tables or chairs.

Effects

Short Wave Diathermy causes increased vascular supply to the treated area which helps to the relaxation of the muscles and thereby the muscle spasm is reduced. Decreased pain perception, increased local metabolism and increased soft tissue extensibility are some of the other effects.

3.6.3.4 ULTRA SOUND THERAPY

Ultrasound is a deep heating modality that uses high-frequency acoustic vibration above the human audible spectrum, defined as frequencies greater than audible sound waves. Ultrasound energy is generated by the piezoelectric effect; electrical energy is applied to a crystal, causing it to vibrate at a high frequency and to produce ultrasound. Ultrasound is delivered by continuous or pulsed wave (the goal is to produce non-thermal effects such as streaming and cavitation) and provides a high heating intensity.